Praise for *Yoga Adjustments*

"As someone who is regularly called upon to treat yoga students injured by ill-informed teachers, I can confidently say that Mark Stephens has done our community a wonderful service with his newest work, *Yoga Adjustments*. Along with *Teaching Yoga* and *Yoga Sequencing*, this book forms a trilogy of essential works for every yoga teacher who strives to be more sensitive, safe, and effective in their teaching."

—**LESLIE KAMINOFF**, founder of The Breathing Project, NYC, and coauthor of *Yoga Anatomy*

"Whether you're in training to be a teacher, just starting your teaching career, or a veteran with many years of experience, Mark Stephens' *Yoga Adjustments* will prove to be an invaluable resource. As with all his work, this book is written with intelligence, insight, and integrity."

—**RICHARD ROSEN**, director of teacher training at Piedmont Yoga and author of *Original Yoga*

"I'm very excited about Mark Stephens' new book, which offers an invaluable service to the yoga community—teachers, aspiring teachers, and yoga students. As yoga's popularity grows, we need our yoga teachers to mature as well, and Mark has given them a superb guidebook for making smart, safe, clear asana adjustments that further our understanding and deepen our experience of yoga. In this way, the benefits of Mark's expertise extend beyond the yoga community by demonstrating how healthy environments can be created in which anybody can practice yoga with confidence."

—**CYNDI LEE**, founder of NYC's Om Yoga and author of *May I Be Happy* and *Yoga Body, Buddha Mind*

"Another monumental and much-needed work to guide yoga teachers in making safe and effective hands-on adjustments with their students. Once again Mark Stephens raises the bar and accelerates the evolutionary path of modern yoga. This book is an invaluable reference for today's and future teachers."

—**GANGA WHITE**, founder and codirector of The White Lotus Foundation and author of *Yoga Beyond Belief*

"This book is an important contribution to the ongoing evolution of yoga teaching and practice. Hands-on adjustments provide a quick and amazing two-way communication stream between teacher and student. Used with or without verbal cues, they can bypass most abstract theory and induce good alignment to reveal how a pose might feel when balanced, open, flowing, and free. Conversely, adjustments can be mechanical and even manipulative, seductive, and harmful. Because of this powerful potential in both ways, we all need to look intelligently at their mechanics, purposes, and ethics. Stephens' *Yoga Adjustments* is a wonderfully detailed resource for our investigation."

—**RICHARD FREEMAN**, director of The Yoga Workshop and author of *The Mirror of Yoga*

"Just as a good massage feels great and is healing, and a bad massage can be annoying, even painful and unpleasant, so it goes with hands-on assists in yoga. May this book encourage healing touch! Thank you, Mark, for making this information so accessible and clear!"

—**ERICH SCHIFFMANN**, founder of Freedom Style Yoga and author of *Yoga: The Spirit and Practice of Moving Into Stillness*

"I love that Mark Stephens has covered not just the biomechanics of hands-on assists and the spectrum from technical support to subtle energetic direction, but also the internal dynamics and ethics that the power of touch brings up in people of all walks of life. Mark offers practical insights, including the many dimensions of respecting a person's process, injuries, and tweaks, and the important boundaries that are necessary for entering this territory that is often like being a 'midwife of the embodied experience.' Mark brings understanding to the somatic power of touch and the role of hands-on assists in the unfolding of yoga. This is a book that will surely be serving teachers for a long time."

> —**SHIVA REA**, founder of Prana Flow®–Energetic Vinyasa and author of *Tending the Heart Fire*

"We generally think of touch as from one person to another. In this book, Stephens reminds us that we must first be 'in touch' with ourselves and with our own yoga practice before adjusting another person's pose. Overall, the book focuses on practical application of adjustments, based on fundamental elements of an ethical personal practice. On asanas, Stephens states that the teacher should understand 'their benefits, risks, contraindications, preparatory asanas, alignment principals, energetic actions, common challenges, modifications, use of props.' Quite thorough, the step-by-step examples are threaded throughout with groundwork in both Western and yoga philosophy. It is a pleasure to read."

> —**LISA WALFORD**, curriculum director of Yoga Works Teacher Training and senior certified Iyengar Yoga teacher

"Finally, the book I have been waiting for—a clear and thorough guide to hands-on assisting in yoga. Mark Stephens takes us from the guiding principles of touch observation of students, and establishing intention for touching, through to specific verbal cues and hands-on instruction to support those cues. For teachers, he offers stances to safely ground ourselves while adjusting a student along with terminology for clarifying the various ways of touching for maximum effectiveness. Additionally, Mark provides clear guidance on how *not* to touch. All of this culminates in a comprehensive index of poses with verbal cues and clear photographs explaining the various options for hands-on assistance to provide greater alignment in the asanas. Never before have we teachers and students had such a concise guide available to us."

> —**MARION (MUGS) McCONNELL**, founder of South Okanagan Yoga Academy, British Columbia

"A must-read for any yoga teacher looking to expand and deepen not only their knowledge of adjustments, but also of teaching asana as well. The level of detail and knowledge presented here is phenomenal."

> —**CHRIS COURTNEY**, yoga teacher and editor-at-large of *Elephant Journal*

Yoga
Adjustments

Also by Mark Stephens

Teaching Yoga: Essential Foundations and Techniques
Yoga Sequencing: Designing Transformative Yoga Classes

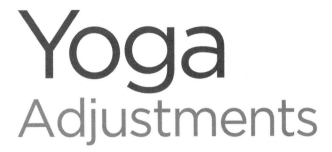

Yoga
Adjustments

PHILOSOPHY, PRINCIPLES, AND TECHNIQUES

MARK STEPHENS

Foreword by Shiva Rea

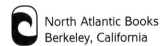
North Atlantic Books
Berkeley, California

Published by
North Atlantic Books
P.O. Box 12327
Berkeley, California 94712

Cover photo by Beau Roulette
Cover and book design by Suzanne Albertson

Printed in the United States of America

Yoga Adjustments: Philosophy, Principles, and Techniques is sponsored by the Society for the Study of Native Arts and Sciences, a nonprofit educational corporation whose goals are to develop an educational and cross-cultural perspective linking various scientific, social, and artistic fields; to nurture a holistic view of arts, sciences, humanities, and healing; and to publish and distribute literature on the relationship of mind, body, and nature.

North Atlantic Books' publications are available through most bookstores. For further information, visit our website at www.northatlanticbooks.com or call 800–733–3000.

Library of Congress Cataloging-in-Publication Data

Stephens, Mark, 1958-
    Yoga adjustments : philosophy, principles, and techniques / Mark Stephens ; foreword by Shiva Rea.
        pages cm
    Includes bibliographical references and index.
    ISBN 978–1-58394–770–8 (alk. paper)—ISBN 978–1-58394–784–5 (ebook)
  1. Hatha yoga. 2. Yoga—Philosophy. I. Title.
    RA781.7.S7275 2014
    613.7'046—dc23   2013027516

1 2 3 4 5 6 7 8 9 SHERIDAN 19 18 17 16 15 14

Printed on recycled paper

To everyone on the path of sustainable and transformational yoga.

CONTENTS

Contents

FOREWORD by Shiva Rea

It is the last evening Vinyasa class at Yoga Works in 1994. In a sea of rhythmic flow and deepening meditation, everybody from all walks of life, shapes, sizes, and levels of experience moves together. In between these whole-body mudras—standing postures that change into back bends, twists, forward bends—there is the guiding intelligence of hands-on assists that follow the flow of breath. The language of touch—the somatic knowing that formed our first way of experiencing the world—gives visceral direction to my guidance by words: "Ground your thighs into the earth." "Lengthen the spine from the base." "Move your shoulder blades into your body." "Reach through the crown of the head." "Feel your heart expand into the space."

Our hands teach the foundation of asana and assist the flow of yoga, reflecting a knowledge and wisdom that applies to life. Where are you coming from? Where are you evolving to? How do you move in a way that is connected to your center? Hands-on assists reveal a potential that is waiting to be embodied. And like life, hands-on assists are sometimes firm and at other times light and subtle, taking us across the places we fear and delivering us into the places we call home.

Back in the day, Mark Stephens was an amazing assistant to my evening classes where there was a palpable magic to the evolving synthesis of the Vinyasa Flow form that I am proud to say twenty-two years later I was instrumental in helping to pioneer and evolve. In these late-night classes, where the mental swirl of urban life surrendered more easily into the nonverbal state of flow, I remember the energy of the room where I would be on one end of the room and Mark on the other, and we would look up and behold the satisfaction of people going deeper in their own embodiment and the quiet power that hands-on assists offers to that process.

I was grateful to be able to share with Mark and the students what had been passed on to me by my teachers at the time—Sri Pattabhi Jois, Chuck Miller, and Erich Schiffmann, who were amazing teachers of the art of transformative assists. The process of giving an "assist" can range from a daily educational grounding and support to the profoundly life-changing. I could see back then in my classes that Mark was absorbing this knowledge, and it is a celebration to be able to offer the foreword to his evolution in this compendium for all teachers on the art of hands-on assisting.

Mark's previous life in academia, as a director of alternative education and as a yoga studio owner, has given him the fortitude, scope, and honest approach to this knowledge, which deserves to be honored for its true complexity and clarity. I love that he has covered not just the biomechanics of hands-on assists and the spectrum from technical support to subtle energetic direction but also the internal dynamics and ethics that the power of touch brings up in people of all walks of life. Mark offers practical dynamics that include the many dimensions of respecting a person's process, injuries, and tweaks as well as the important boundaries that are necessary for entering this territory that is often like being a "midwife of the embodied experience." Mark brings understanding to the somatic power of touch and the role of hands-on assists in the unfolding of yoga.

Like Mark's previous book on sequencing, he is making accessible the many layers of this knowledge from across different schools of yoga, which is a real accomplishment. I especially appreciate how he continues to underline the importance of really knowing the dynamics of an asana in your own body—its key actions, *vinyasa krama* (stages of practice), and contraindications—before giving effective assists.

Thank you, Mark, for your time and effort in providing this service for yoga teachers everywhere. As I am writing this in the midst of finishing my first book, I can appreciate the tremendous dedication it takes to transfer living knowledge into the written form. I feel in your writing the same qualities that I first recognized in you back in those evening classes. You show up for life fully and are willing to do your own work and open to the full process of yoga in your own evolution. Congratulations for completing this offering to the yoga world—a book that will surely be serving teachers for a long time.

May all beings who embark upon this journey open to the power of embodiment through yoga and the gift within our hands for awareness, healing, support, and integration.

Sarva Mangalam—Auspiciousness for all.

—Shiva Rea
Founder of Prana Flow® Energetic Vinyasa

PREFACE

This book is for anyone on the yoga teaching path who is committed to teaching classes that are safe, sustainable, and transformational. With over 100,000 yoga teachers in North America alone and new yoga teacher-training programs opening nearly every day, the ranks of the yoga teaching profession are growing proportionately more quickly than the increase in students taking yoga classes. While one might be tempted to see this as a boon to students looking for the right teacher, there is legitimate concern over the core competencies of teachers who themselves might be beginning yoga students or otherwise limited in yoga experience or knowledge. Long gone are the days when most teachers studied and apprenticed for many years or even decades under the guidance of a highly experienced mentor, and the mentoring days may be limited for those veteran mentor teachers who are not keeping pace with the many advancements and refinements in the techniques and methods of teaching yoga, especially amid concerted efforts to elevate yoga teaching to a bona fide and widely respected profession marked by high standards of training and competence.

When writing my first book for yoga teachers, *Teaching Yoga: Essential Foundations and Techniques,* my focus was on offering a broad text covering all of the main elements of teaching yoga, including yoga history and philosophy, subtle energy and the highlights of functional anatomy, general techniques and methods for teaching asana classes, how to teach various *pranayama* and meditation techniques, and the basics of sequencing and working with specialized needs among students. Meanwhile, as I peered more closely at how teachers were designing their classes and listened to teachers discussing their greatest challenges, I was inspired to write *Yoga Sequencing: Designing Transformative Yoga Classes.* That second book for teachers addresses a simple question at the heart of teaching sensible yoga classes: *why this, then that?* It presents the philosophy, principles, and techniques for designing yoga classes, looks closely at how to sequence one's instructional cues, offers sixty-seven model sequences for a wide variety of student needs and intensions, and practical resources for sensibly designing one's own unique yoga classes.

Just as that second book was going to press, the bombshell of William J. Broad's provocative article on "How Yoga Can Wreck Your Body" appeared in the *New York Times.* Like many others in the yoga community, my reaction to Broad's statements was as swift as it was visceral; it felt like he was hitting the yoga community below the belt, and I, like many others, passionately responded in writing. I also reached out to Broad directly to try to better understand his concerns and his sources. He sent me a massive database on yoga-related injuries compiled through the National Consumer Product Safety Commission's National Electronic Injury Surveillance System (NEISS). Although I find some of that data contains ecological fallacies or other issues of integrity, Broad's basic message—that doing yoga can wreck your body—is well supported by it.[1] Looking more closely at that data, at Broad's subsequent book, *The Science of Yoga,* and many similar articles published in the popular press over the past twenty years, but also listening to the stories of innumerable teachers confused by even very basic student conditions, the need for the present book became abundantly clear.[2]

This book is all about the nuances of teaching asanas and making them as accessible and sustainable as can be for the real human beings doing them in our classes. In teaching asanas, we rely primarily on three means of conveying guidance to our students: visual demonstration, verbal cues, and tactile cues. To the extent that you as the teacher are clear in understanding what you are attempting to communicate to the student, any of these three methods can effectively lead a student to adjust and refine what he or she is doing in a way that makes that student's practice more safe, sustainable, and transformational. This is the primary mantra of this book: *safe, sustainable, transformational.* Here we look at the balanced and appropriate use of these means of guidance, giving close attention to how they are uniquely interrelated in guiding any particular asana.

Our purpose as yoga teachers is to guide and inspire students in their personal practice, ultimately to a place where the student can continue practicing through his or her life guided by the best teacher they will ever have—the one inside. This involves a relationship between teacher and student that is open, clear, and respectful. Our role as teachers is not to give forceful adjustments that somehow correct postural forms, nor to assist students in going far beyond what they are capable of on their own. We are at best informed and inspiring guides, ideally informed by knowledge of the terrain, the conditions and intentions of our students, and perhaps something greater that inspires you to fully devote yourself to sharing this practice in meaningful ways.

In my own evolution and learning along the yoga path, I've been very lucky to have diversely insightful teachers whose depth of personal commitment to the practice and to the art and science of transmitting it to others was not only contagious but was a primary source of the foundational knowledge presented here. My first yoga teacher, Erich Schiffmann, taught me how to relate hands-on adjustments to the principles of alignment and energetic actions in the asanas. Chuck Miller taught me how to give assistance amid the flowing set sequences of Ashtanga Vinyasa. Jasmine Lieb, with whom I apprenticed for six months, shared with me her keen insights into teaching beginning-level students as well as those with a variety of physical challenges—insights she received from training with Indra Devi, through her practice, and through her physical therapy background. After crossing paths with Shiva Rea in Ashtanga Vinyasa classes, Iyengar workshops, and in her own pioneering Vinyasa Flow classes in the early 1990s, I assisted her in classes, workshops, and on retreats in which she revealed some of the powerfully inspirational ways that a teacher can share the practice in syncopation with the rhythms and seasons of life. Many others have influenced me through workshops in further developing the skills and insights that I have synthesized, expanded, refined, and presented here: Kofi Busia, Tim Miller, Lisa Walford, Dona Holleman, Rodney Yee, Judith Lasater, Ramanand Patel, Richard Freeman, Patricia Walden, participants in my hands-on adjustments workshops over the past fifteen years, and amazing students who have always been my most insightful teachers. I am grateful to all.

In crafting this book, I once again had the joy of working with the folks at North Atlantic Books, many of whom are very much on the yoga path or kindred spirits in exploring consciousness and becoming. Doug Reil encouraged me to devote myself to this project when at times I considered other ideas, offering several suggestions that helped me craft the book as it is. My project editor, Leslie Larson, guided the entire process of moving from a manuscript to a published book. Christopher Church once again made my writing clearer and helped bring greater coherence to the manuscript. Suzanne Albertson's cover and inside book design beautifully speaks for itself.

Several friends, colleagues, and fellow teachers provided invaluable comments on various drafts of my original manuscript: Anne Tharpe, Daniel Stewart, Darren

Main, Elise Oliphant, Ganga White, Joanna Bechuza, Karen Dunn, Max Tarjan, Megan Burke, Melinda Bukey, Richard Rosen, Sean Lang, Sarah Finney, and Todd Tuholke.

Several of my students and teacher-training graduates patiently modeled for the asana photographs: Amy Hsiung, Andreas Kahl, Anne Tharpe, Erika Abrahamian, Jennifer Lung, Marcia Charland, Max Tarjan (cover), Michelle Naklowycz, Nadia Lewis (cover), Pat Tao, Ray Charland, Samantha Rae Boozer, Sean Lang, Shannon McQuaide, and Tom Simpkins. James Wvinner shot all the asana and hands-on adjustments photos.

This book would not have been possible without the loving support of DiAnna Van Eycke, Melinda Bukey, Michael Stephens, Jennifer Stanley, Mike Rotkin, James Wvinner, Ralph Quinn, Siddha, and Pi.

Part I
Foundations

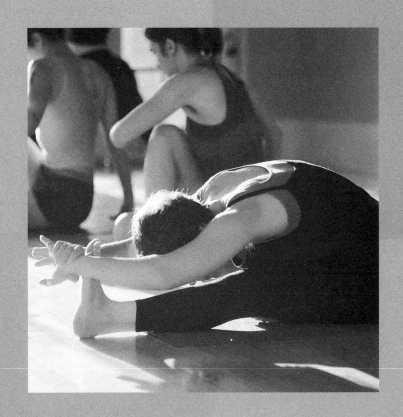

Chapter 1

Philosophy and Sensibility in Giving Yoga Adjustments

PART OF THE SUBLIME NATURE OF YOGA IS THAT there are infinite possibilities for deepening and refining one's practice. In playing the edges of effort and ease, exploring balance between surrender and control, and opening to self-understanding and self-transformation, there is no end to how far one can go along the path of awakening to clearer awareness, more integrated well-being, and greater happiness. There are also seemingly infinite styles and approaches to yoga, even different ideas about what yoga is, offering a rich array of practices that any of the seven billion of us sharing this planet might at any given time find most in keeping with whatever brings us to explore this ancient ritual for living in the most healthy and awakened way. It's a fascinating, challenging, often mysterious path that ultimately reveals the deepest beauty inherent in each of us as we gradually come to discover the balances that most complement and support our diverse values and intentions in life. If along the path one becomes a teacher—a guide on the yoga path—then the practice itself blossoms even more as practicing and guiding each bring light to the other.

In doing yoga, the best teacher one will ever have is alive and well inside. In every breath, every posture, and all the moments and transitions in between, the inner teacher is offering guidance. The tone, texture, and tempo of the breath blend with myriad sensations arising in the bodymind to suggest how and where one might best go with focused awareness and action.[1] There is no universally correct method or technique, no set of rules, no single goal, and no absolute authority beyond what comes to the practitioner through the heart and soul of simply being in it, listening inside, and opening to the possibilities of amazing qualities of being fully, consciously alive. It's a personal practice, even if one comes to it and finds in it a more abiding sense of social connection or spiritual being.[2]

Yet there is inestimable value and purpose in having outer teachers and in teaching yoga. While with consistent and refined practice students develop the awareness that makes the asanas more understandable, accessible, and sustainable from the inside out, gradually and more clearly feeling their way into sequences that work, nearly all of us benefit from the informed insights of a trained and experienced teacher whose guidance, even just on matters of postural alignment and energetic actions, can make our experience in doing yoga safer and more beneficial. A teacher can also give guidance on techniques and qualities of breathing, mental attentiveness, postural modifications and variations, sequences within and between asana families, as well as adaptations to address special conditions such as frailty, tightness, hypermobility, pregnancy, and interrelated physical, physiological, and psychological pathologies. Put differently, teachers matter; the question is, how do we best teach?

As yoga teachers, we employ a variety of techniques to support and guide our students, including through the spirited or charismatic ways we generally hold the space of a class, the use of physical demonstration, verbal cues, even metaphor and stories to add inspiration and insight. Each of these aspects of teaching involves tapping into all of our inner resources along with ongoing learning and practice. With time and consistent presence on the path of the teacher, these qualities become more integrated into our evolving repertoire of knowledge and skills that enable us as teachers to guide student practices in a way that makes sense for the actual students in our immediate presence—this in contrast to teaching in a cookie-cutter fashion as if everyone were the same and the same exact practice made sense for all of humanity.

There is no end to how much we can learn and evolve as teachers. True to the maxim posited by the Greek philosopher Aristotle that "the more you know, the more you know you don't know,"[3] the further you go in your training, learning, and experience as a yoga teacher, the more you'll realize that there's an infinite universe of knowledge and wisdom to bring to the practice. This becomes more abundantly clear as we come to better appreciate and understand our students, which is absolutely essential if we are to guide them well in their practice. To get a better sense of this, let's look at the practice itself and the basic elements and sensibilities of teaching.

Unique Students, Unique Teaching

We all come to the practice of yoga uniquely. While we are all human beings, that's where the uniformity ends, because we're a beautifully diverse species with different genetic endowments, life experiences, lifestyles, conditions, and intentions. Consider for a moment these examples of differences:

- A thirty-five-year-old mother of two with a background in dance and surgically repaired anterior cruciate ligaments who sits for long hours working as a financial analyst.
- A twenty-three-year-old pregnant astrophysics graduate student in peak athletic condition and with bipolar disorder.
- A fifty-four-year-old Buddhist nun with a thirty-year consistent yoga practice and advanced osteoporosis.
- A twenty-year-old college student with a pronounced right thoracic scoliosis.
- A sixty-one-year-old recently retired software engineer with years of weight training and extremely tight muscles who is recovering from breast cancer.
- A forty-one-year-old beginning yoga teacher free of injuries who proudly enjoys showing off his gymnastic ability in the front of class.

Welcome to the reality of teaching yoga. If you intend to teach public yoga classes where it's anyone's guess who might show up, you should anticipate having a diverse array of students, student conditions, and student intentions in your classes: serious students for whom yoga practice is essential to daily life in healing traumas and purely athletic weekend warriors; spiritual seekers and people of strong religious faith as well as those for whom faith is seen as intellectual weakness; every age, every interest, every philosophical perspective, and every condition.

Given the vast differences among students, it's important to give guidance that addresses unique conditions while teaching in a way that makes sense for the entire class. (Ideally students go to classes that are appropriate for them; just don't count on it, but do count on diversity.) So before getting even close to matters of hands-on guidance and adjustments (as well as other means of providing guidance), there are other qualities to emphasize in helping to ensure that students practice in keeping with the realities of their lives.

The Heart of Practicing and Guiding Yoga

At the risk of stating the obvious, in practicing yoga we all start from where we are—this in contrast to where someone else might think we are or where we ourselves might mistakenly think we are. Many teachers have preconceived or ill-informed ideas about the abilities or interests of their students while many students over- or underestimate their immediately present ability. How as teachers might we best navigate these realities? By guiding our students to cultivate a personal practice that reflects their own values, intentions, and conditions, even as these all may (and likely will) evolve.

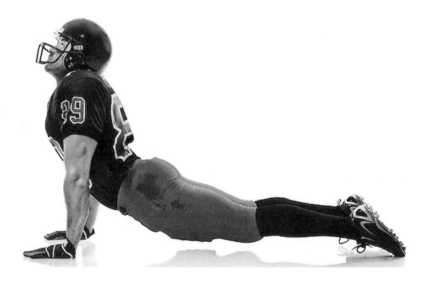

Doing yoga is a personal practice, not a competitive sport.

There are several basic elements that are ideally communicated to our students in every practice and given even greater clarity with newer students.[4] Among the most important is the idea that yoga is neither a comparative nor a competitive practice, despite some people doing their best to make it so.[5] Exploring with this basic sensibility, the practice will be more safe, sustainable, and transformational. It's a sensibility—a basic yogic value—that reflects the sole comment on asana found in the oft-cited Yoga Sutras of Patanjali: *sthira, sukham, asanam*—meaning steadiness, ease, and presence of mind (the latter, from the root word *as,* meaning "to take one seat," which I interpret to mean to be here now, fully attuned to one's immediate experience). It's helpful to relate to these as qualities we're always cultivating in the practice. Do note that Patanjali is not describing anything even closely approximating the sort of postural practices that began evolving several hundred years later and eventually became Hatha yoga, which has evolved more in the past seventy-five years than in the previous thousand.[6] Nonetheless, we find the sensibilities of classical yoga brought forward in the earliest verified writing on Hatha practice, the mid-fourteenth-century *Hatha Yoga Pradipika,* where Swami Swatmarama tells the yogi to have "enthusiasm, perseverance, discrimination, unshakable faith, courage" to "bring success to yoga" and "get steadiness of body and mind." Later, Swatmarama (1985, 54, 67, 132) mentions "being free of fatigue in practicing asana," suggesting the balance of steadiness and ease earlier emphasized by Patanjali.

Exploring this, let's say for a moment that we're starting a practice standing at the front of the mat (bearing in mind here that the same concepts, qualities, and sensibilities are ideally cultivated regardless of one's initial postural position—sitting, lying supine, and so on). This standing posture might be called Tadasana (Mountain Pose). In it, we're opening to being as steady, at ease, and present as can be—imagine a mountain!—and thereby more naturally opening to a deepening sense of balance and equanimity that is well expressed with another Sanskrit term: *samasthihi* (literally, "equal standing"). For some students, this simple position is somewhat challenging, especially if held for several minutes or if a student has a condition such as general postural misalignment, advanced pregnancy, multiple sclerosis, leg length discrepancy, or basic weakness. With practice, it's likely to become easier to find and sustain a sense of samasthihi in this position, especially with proper alignment and energetic actions. If all one did was to continue standing and moving into deeper equanimity (or sitting or lying supine), this might become more of a meditation practice. But here we are primarily on the path of asana, the postural practices that are best explored with conscious breathing and presence of mind (the reciprocal effects of which we will discuss below as further essential aspects of asana practice).[7]

As we come to the experience in an asana in which we no longer feel any significant effect or effort in being in it, we might simply stay there, being in it, or we might find ourselves opening to a variation of it or transitioning to an asana in which we find it takes some greater effort to find stability and ease to be just as stable, relaxed, and present. However, if we always practice asanas in a way that involves no effort—that is one path—we might be missing an opportunity to engender deeper awakening and change through the intensity and diversity of experience that doing yoga offers us, to really do Hatha yoga, which is most deeply and lastingly done with the self-discipline (*tapas*) it takes to fully show up to the best of our ability, breath by breath, asana by asana, practice by practice, day by day, exploring the edges of possibility and discovering what happens amid it all. With persevering practice—*abhyasa*—we do stay with it; fully committed to the practice, we proceed with deeper experience and reflection, opening to and learning from the intensity of the experience each breath of the way.

This involves staying close to the edges of possibility in what we're doing in our practice, an approach Joel Kramer, a pioneering innovator of contemporary yoga who significantly influenced the evolution of the practice in the 1960s and 1970s, beautifully and richly describes. As we begin moving into an asana, we come to a place where we feel something starting to happen, what Kramer (1977) calls "the primary edge" (I call it the "aha moment").[8] Going further, we come to another "edge" where the bodymind expresses pain, discomfort, or simply blocks further range of motion (I call it the "uh-uh moment"). In a persevering practice, we "play the edge" by staying beyond the "aha" but well enough within the "uh-uh" to have the space to slowly and patiently explore small refining intentional movements. Breath by breath, the edges tend to move—we open more space and create more sustainable ease, thus more easily moving awakening energy throughout the bodymind. If right up against the final edge of possibility or if moving too quickly, there is no space or time for this sense-based refinement and awakening; instead we're likely to cause injury, reinforce unhealthy habits, or simply burn out on the practice.

As much as fully showing up in the practice and playing the edges of possibility and refinement are essential in doing yoga, there's another essential quality of the practice, what Patanjali gives as *vairagya*—nonattachment. In the practice of nonattachment we open to being in the practice with a sense that anything is possible, with spontaneity yet still with self-disciplined effort, all the while identifying more with the deeper intention in our heart—perhaps health, contentment, happiness—than with the performance of a pose or attainment of some static or predetermined goal. Abhyasa and vairagya are thus integrally interrelated elements of a safe, sustainable, and transformational yoga practice that allow us to progress from one place to another with steadiness and ease. Together they give us one of the most basic yogic principles: *it's not about how far you go, but how you go.*

Cueing students in the asanas with a balanced attitude of vairagya and abhyasa helps ensure that they feel supported in their practice while feeling free of attainment-related expectation. By conveying this attitude through every aspect of one's teaching, including in offering and giving tactile cues, students more naturally find their way to their inner teacher, utilizing the intensity of physical sensation and the barometer of the breath to guide their effort in their personal practice.

Indeed, an essential element of this balanced approach to sustainable and transformational yoga practice rests in the breath. Curiously, although the classical writings on Hatha yoga give primary emphasis to pranayama (from *pra*, "to bring forth," *an*, "to breathe," and a combination of *ayama*, "to expand," and *yama*, "to control"), pranayama practice—basic yogic breathing—is typically given little attention in many contemporary yoga classes.[9] As with asana practice, with pranayama it's important to develop the practice gradually and with steadiness and ease.[10] However, soft, gentle, subtle *ujjayi*—"uplifting"—pranayama can be safely practiced by all, including complete beginners, pregnant women, and those with blood-pressure issues, infirmities, and other pathological conditions. The breath itself nourishes our cells and our entire being. The light sound of ujjayi helps us keep our awareness in the breath in a way that makes it easier to cultivate the smooth, balanced, steady flow of each and every inhalation and exhalation, providing immediate feedback on our movement in, through, and out of the asanas. As such, it is a perfect barometer for sensing and cultivating energetic balance in doing asana practices. If the breath is strained, it's a sure sign that one has slipped away from steadiness and ease. Rather than trying to squeeze the breath into the asanas and the movements within and between them, ideally our practice finds expression in and through the integrity of the breath. As we will see, this is equally an essential element in guiding the practice. As we move closer to crossing the bridge from practicing to teaching yoga, all of these qualities of practice become part of the path of the teacher.

In bringing these elements of practice more alive in all of one's teaching techniques and methods, the key is to approach our students in a way that helps them to move more stably, easily, and joyfully in the wise progression of their personal practice. One aspect of this is in how we arrange our classes. In teaching yoga classes, we ideally create an arc-like structure with specific asanas sequenced in a way that makes them accessible, safe, and sustainable—and thereby more deeply transformational.[11] Along the practice path it's helpful to move from simple to more complex postures, generally warming the body while giving focused attention to areas where one will soon explore and go more deeply. Anticipatory asanas open and stabilize the muscles and joints most involved in the peak, helping to further awaken the deeper embodied intelligence one will tap into when exploring the deeper, more complex peak asanas.

This approach reflects the concept of vinyasa krama, from *vinyasa,* "to place in a special way," and *krama,* "stage," referring to the effective sequencing of actions. The essence of vinyasa krama is the wisdom of gradual progression, exploring and evolving consciously and methodically, moving steadily and simply from where one is to wherever one is going with the integrated qualities of abhyasa and vairagya. In bringing fuller integration to this practice, we do *pratikriyasana,* from *prati,* "opposite," and *kriya,* "action," methodically and creatively resolving whatever tension arises along the path leading to Savasana (Corpse Pose) and beyond with compensatory asanas. Breath by breath, we evolve in and through the practice.

Crossing the Bridge from Practicing to Guiding

When doing a yoga practice, we come to various asanas. In approaching them, we're already experiencing sensations. If we're actually doing yoga rather than merely exercising, then we're breathing consciously and using the breath to refine how we're exploring the asana. Breathing consciously, we're bringing more conscious awareness into the bodymind, ideally as suggested by the sensations that are arising in the moment, adapting our movement and positioning to be more stable, relaxed, and present. So there's a dance of the breath with the bodymind, each affecting the other, all of it increasingly experienced as part of the whole of our being. This is the basic practice of always and forever integrating and awakening that is at the heart of yoga asana practice. In it, we can play with different breathing techniques, positions, and visualizations, exploring their various effects, including the inner dialogue and reactions that are an increasingly clear reflective mirror of our deeper qualities of being.

In communicating with our students to convey insights about how they might best approach and explore their practice in a way that reflects and embodies the principles of steadiness and ease, perseverance and nonattachment, we can tap into a variety of resources—speaking, demonstrating, touching, and for some even singing to evoke the spirit of being fully in this self-reflective and potentially transformational practice. The specific combination of techniques we use in any given situation ideally reflects both our personal sensibilities and our best sense of how the students we're teaching might best explore and learn in keeping with their own intentions and sensibilities. Indeed, how people learn is closely tied to what Howard Gardner (1993) refers to as "qualities of multiple intelligence," which vary considerably in any given class. Some students learn well from verbal messages while others need a visual model in order to "get it" in their bodymind. Still others are primarily tactile or kinematic learners: they need to feel it in order to most fully comprehend it internally. In yoga classes, where the learning experience includes conceptual, emotional, physical, and spiritual elements, this full range of learning styles is always at play.

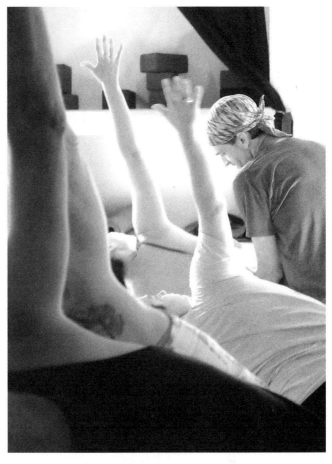

While the best yoga teacher one will ever have is alive and well inside, the outer teacher's role can help students discover their inner teacher.

At the same time, a human being is more than the sum of her or his intellectual or intuitive tendencies; motivation, personality, emotions, physical health, and personal will are often more significant than a particular learning style in shaping how, where, and when one learns. This suggests that effective yoga instruction should address these differences while engaging with students in a way that appreciates and honors the rich variety of learning styles. With hands-on yoga teaching, we can work with students to guide, refine, and support their developing practices beyond the expressions and limitations of the spoken word and visual demonstration. Put differently, the beautiful diversity of conditions, intentions, and learning styles suggests the value of a richly varied and nuanced approach to teaching.

Guiding with Your Hands

Using your hands to accentuate and refine what you are trying to convey with words or visual modeling can make all the difference in a student's ability to comprehend and internalize whatever you are trying to share. (When discussing hands-on adjustments, guidance, assisting, touch, and so on, we're using *hands-on* in both the general and specific meaning of the term—the general referring to tactile guidance that might involve using one's hands, arms, shoulders, torso, hips, legs, or feet, and the specific referring to the hands. Unless specifically indicated, the use of the term refers to its general meaning.) With clearer, more manifold communication comes deeper learning, and with it the promise of yoga—to be healthy, integrated, fully awake—is gradually more fully realized. Touch, which immediately reaches our students in a direct and personal way, can thus be an effective method of directly, simply, and specifically communicating with them.[12]

Spoken words and the physical demonstration of asanas are essential ways of communicating with students and should be the starting place—and often the ending place—in teaching asanas. Yet when combined with precise and informed touch, these tools can convey even more:

- clarifying a verbalized or demonstrated alignment cue
- highlighting an energetic action
- giving students a feeling of support
- bringing awareness to an unconscious part of the body
- assisting in stabilizing, easing, or deepening an asana
- assisting in safely increasing range of motion
- helping you as the teacher to be more aware of a student's overall condition
- creating a more trusting and open sense of connection between you and your students
- offering comforting support amid the intensity of some experiences

Yet while touch is among the most profoundly effective tools in teaching and learning yoga, it can also be among the most potentially problematic. Giving tactile guidance should help students in developing a safe, sustainable, and transformational practice, but done wrong, it can cause physical or emotional harm. Given with clear and informed intention, hands-on cues can clarify other ways of guiding students, while ill-informed hands-on cues can confuse students in feeling their way into and refining an asana. Offered appropriately, students will learn to trust their inner teacher, while if given excessively, physical cues can make a student dependent on an external source of guidance and distract him or her from the tapas element—self-discipline—in doing yoga. Hands-on guidance can also be a source of greater openness, inspiration, and joy, yet can cause discomfort, trauma, or disillusion with yoga if a teacher's cues convey judgment or violate personal boundaries.

The primary purpose of tactile cues is to help students refine their yoga practice as a personal process for cultivating wellness, self-discovery, and self-transformation. Yet yoga practice is ultimately an internal process that is best guided from inside through the intertwined prisms of the breath and awareness in the bodymind.[13] As teachers, we can best assist our students by helping them learn to listen inside and honor their inner teacher, offering hands-on guidance only when it's both welcome and beneficial to the student. Doing this well starts by embracing the idea of teaching people who are doing asanas, not poses.[14]

Poses are static representations of idealized forms, something models do for cameras in an effort to send an external message. Typically airbrushed and enhanced in other ways, they are anything but real. Asanas, by contrast, are alive and personal; they are an expression of organic human beings exploring, living,

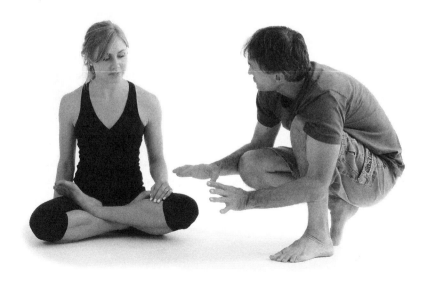

Always appreciate that you are teaching people, not poses.

and intentionally evolving in the temple of the bodymind. When we appreciate a student through the wisdom of our heart, then we more naturally see the intrinsic beauty already manifest in their practice. From this starting point we come to more naturally sit in the seat of the teacher, giving our students the space to blossom in the fullness of their yoga—even when we apply what insight we might have into the basic architecture, gesture, and mood of each asana as it is uniquely and beautifully expressed in each individual student.

In giving tactile cues, we are offering students guidance in finding their way to a more stable foundation, to aligning their body safely and comfortably, and to encouraging deeper exploration while staying connected to the breath and bodymind as their principal sources of guidance. We are guiding our students on a journey set primarily by each student's own intention, whether sensed as physical, emotional, mental, or spiritual. When we approach and guide students with this attitude, it empowers them to go as deeply as they are meant to go in that moment of their practice, further clarifies the teacher-student relationship, and reinforces an open-minded and open-hearted experience in doing yoga. In this relationship, yoga teachers are engaging in a quality of social interaction that forms an important part of the environment of the student's yoga practice and sense of being, and in this relationship, both teacher and student are transformed. Let's explore this more deeply, stepping slightly back in order to go more clearly forward.

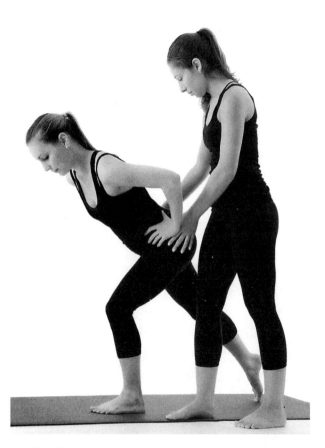

Tactile cues are an integral part of teaching in most approaches to Hatha yoga.

Styles That Touch

The role of touch varies widely across the many styles and traditions of Hatha yoga. Tactile guidance and support is seen as an essential tool in Kripalu, Svaroopa, Phoenix Rising, Viniyoga, and other largely healing or otherwise thera-peutic approaches to yoga.[15] It is also used extensively in Ashtanga Vinyasa, Iyengar, and most Vinyasa Flow, yet is virtually absent in Bikram, YogaFit, and a few other styles.

It is possible to teach any style of yoga with or without tactile guidance and support. Recognizing that the world of yoga is constantly evolving, cross-fertilizing, and diversifying, most yoga teachers will discover that there is a strong likelihood that their own approach will evolve, and that the knowledge and skills for giving appropriate and effective adjustments is likely to be an increasingly important part of one's repertoire as a yoga teacher as one moves farther along the teaching path.

Touch, Somatics, and Self-Transformation

Whether one seeks the meaning or purpose of yoga from ancient texts such as the Bhagavad Gita, Yoga Sutras of Patanjali, or Hatha Yoga Pradipika, or looks to more modern or contemporary sources for guidance and inspiration, awakening to or cultivating clearer awareness, more awakened being, and a better, healthier life are constants. Standing on the edge of the mythical battlefield of the Mahabharata War, Prince Arjuna was frozen in inaction due to misunderstanding the nature of his being; in finding his path *(dharma)*, he would become clearer in his awareness and thereby able to act more consciously and forthrightly in his life.[16] Patanjali similarly identifies the source of human suffering *(klesha)* that motivates yoga in ignorance of one's true nature *(avidya)* that is rooted in a confused bodymind, offering an eight-step approach to betterment that includes moral and personal observances, asana, pranayama, *pratyahara* (relieving the senses of their external distractions), and meditation as a defined path to blissful being *(samadhi)*. Eleven hundred years later—in the mid-fourteenth century CE—Swatmarama elabo-rated a specific regimen of self-purification techniques to be followed sequentially by asana (he describes fifteen, mostly sitting), pranayama, mudra, and bandha practices designed to enhance health, curtail mental confusion, and open to liberation *(moksha)*.

Seemingly a world away, the Greek philosopher Plato pleaded for "an equal and healthy balance between [body and mind]" as his teacher Socrates, who said "no citizen has a right to be an amateur in the matter of physical training. . . . What a disgrace it is for a man to grow old without ever seeing the beauty and strength of which his body is capable," trained in dance to refine his bodymind in keeping with the embodied philosophical practice of the time.[17] "Even in the act of thinking," Socrates affirmed, "which is supposed to require least assistance from the body, everyone knows that serious mistakes happen through physical ill-health." While imbued with a dualist perspective consonant with the dualism found in classical yoga that posits the material world as an illusion (*maya* in the Vedas and Upanishads, "ideal forms" in Plato's thinking), we no less find here the path to a clearer, freer, happier, better life through body-mind integration, clarification, and transformation practices.

Here we'll briefly skim a little more deeply into these questions of philosophy and embodiment, which you might find bring more light to our main topic—guiding the practice. Most of the ensuing development of Western philosophy would deny the importance of the physical realm.[18] Yet by the late nineteenth century we begin to find recognition that embodied intelligence matters in understanding one's experience and in improving one's life. The pragmatist philosopher and pioneering psychologist William James (1976, 86; 1890, 306–11) affirmed the body's pervasive influence on awareness and the bodily dimension of thought and emotion, even if in keeping with the Western dualist tradition that situated the ultimate source of consciousness outside the organic human being. In his view, we do embody experience, and the meliorative project of pragmatic philosophy and psychology—to make life better—must address how emotion and thought are inextricably interwoven in our tissues and expressed in every aspect of bodily posture and language.

The American philosopher and educator John Dewey (2008a, 29–30) drew from James's thinking and went farther in advocating the integration of the body-mind in experiential ways as "the most practical question we can ask of our civilization." Offering a holistic perspective in a spiritual and philosophical universe dominated by dualist thinking and various forms of theological predeterminism in which an autonomous ego or supernatural force manifests everything, Dewey boldly charted a different path, asserting that we have real choices in our lives—even if the realities of our lives are powerfully conditioned by habits of being that in traditional yoga philosophy are explained as *"samskaras"* inherited from past lives and embodied in the totality of our being. "Habits," Dewey (2008b, 21–22) writes, "are demands for certain kinds of activity," the predisposition of which are "an immensely more intimate and fundamental part of ourselves than are vague, general, conscious choices."

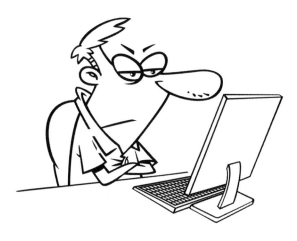

"Mr. Duffy lived at some distance from his body." –James Joyce, *Ulysses*

Put differently, Dewey builds upon and moves beyond James's idea that mental and emotional life are embodied by fully situating consciousness in the bodymind even as it is conditioned by its environmental context, including social forces, giving us the idea of reflective body consciousness that is open to constant evolution through deliberate effort.[19] He calls for "conscious practice" not in pursuit of an idealized notion of some primordial being or transcendence of our present being, but in the reality of this being, right here and now. Dewey's exploration of this in a daily practice, as taught to him by Frederick M. Alexander, of Alexander Technique fame, focused on recognizing and releasing habitual, unhealthy, self-limiting patterns in the bodymind.

Here we take a different path: Hatha yoga in the twenty-first century. The evolution of one's awareness is an integral aspect of yoga as a transformative practice. In Hatha yoga—the big umbrella over all styles, brands, and lineages utilizing postural and movement techniques—this practice is one of more fully awakening and deeply integrating on the path to a more holistic, congruent, and healthy life. Put differently, doing yoga is a practice for awakening to our embodiment as organic humans that happens the moment one becomes present to the experience of breathing and being in this bodymind. For many this is and always will be a spiritual path that is about "being in" (a oneness perspective) or "connecting to" (a dualist perspective) a sense of the infinite or consciousness beyond the bodymind, perhaps (or perhaps not) as a path to transcendence. For others, even if not specifically describing yoga, it's about fully awakening to the spirit and reality of being alive, finding meaning, as Mark Johnson (1989, 10) proposes, "within the flow of experience that cannot exist without a biological organism engaging its environment." Rather than human thought and experience being essentially illusional or somehow "cut off from the world," Johnson (1989, 271–78) points us toward an "embodied, experiential view of meaning" expressed through this "phenomenal body"—not the folk concept of the body that is reduced to biological functioning, but one in which the bodymind is whole.[20] Doing yoga gives us the opportunity to directly experience and cultivate this sense of wholeness in the full reality of our lives in this world.

Relating this approach to practicing and teaching yoga, we are tapping into the concept of somatics. From the Greek *soma,* meaning "living, aware, bodily person," somatics assumes that we are, in our essence, whole beings rather than having the body-mind split that is pervasive in Western philosophy and medicine as well as Eastern spiritual philosophies and metaphysics and which typically places the source of consciousness outside of the organic human. Originally drawing on the pioneering work of William James and Wilhelm Reich, a rich array of practices aimed at holistic bodymind awareness have developed in the field of somatics, including the Feldenkrais Method, Hanna Somatic Education, Ideokinesis, Bodymind Centering, Postural Integration, Rolfing and Trager Approach.[21] As with Dewey's practice of Alexander Technique, these and other somatic practice methods start from the assumption that emotional and mental experience is embodied rather than residing only in the gray matter of the brain or somehow separate from the body. Embodied emotional and mental complexes are seen in turn as causing or exacerbating physical dysfunction or pathology, blocking the full inner manifestation of what Reich referred to as Life Force, a concept of the breath similar to yoga's *prana.* Indeed, much of somatics is consonant with yoga as a practice of self-transformation, starting with the idea of psychic adhesions (yoga's samskaras) blocking healthy awakening on the path to clear awareness (yoga's samadhi).

In the view of somatics, self-transformation must address how to release accumulated tension and thereby bring embodied experience more fully to one's awareness in a way that allows gradual integration of one's life. Somatics typically uses hands-on techniques, including deep-tissue manipulation aimed at releasing deeply held tension. Much of this work uses physical stimulation or manipulation in specific areas of the body to highlight stress responses in which the sympathetic nervous system—the fight-or-flight response—is activated. Using specific breathing techniques—some are similar to ujjayi, *kapalabhati,* and *bastrika* pranayamas—one then gradually brings more subtle awareness to the overall experience of living in the fullness of one's sensations in the bodymind and with it a deeper calm as the parasympathetic nervous system is activated.

Yoga Practice and Teaching Revisited

Let's now bring this back to yoga practice and teaching. Much of the somatics field is concerned with emotional trauma and related therapies. Much of the contemporary yoga scene eschews such work in favor of yoga as glorified or romanticized exercise. Yet yoga originated as, and has always had as its principle focus, a practice of self-transformation into clearer awareness or spiritual being, what for some promises transcendence beyond mortal being. In the Yoga Sutras of Patanjali, this is stated as *citta vrtti nirodaha,* "to calm the fluctuations of the mind" that are seen as the source of ignorance of the reality of one's true being and thus the proximate cause of existential suffering.[22] While Patanjali's approach to yoga does not involve doing asana practice beyond sitting, he offers a yoga psychology that first describes the condition of the confused mind and then a set of actions—a yoga technology—one can undertake to cultivate a clear and healthy mind. As discussed earlier, several hundred years later, Hatha yogis elaborated a system of postural practices, breathing techniques, and mudras designed as a simpler path to same goal, albeit along a path of fuller integration of breath and bodymind, and with it the blossoming of the clear consciousness promised by Patanjali's method.

Part of the beauty of yoga asana practice is that each and every different asana highlights tension and other sensation in the body. Paying closer attention, we also come to detect how the different asanas stimulate different emotional and mental reactions; a certain posture done in a particular way, time, or other circumstance tends to generate its own somewhat unique effects on the mind. Each asana also tends to affect the breath in different ways, however subtle the differences may be. Staying with the breath as we feel it in the body, we

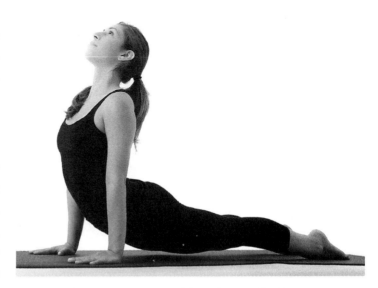

Breathing through the heart in Urdhva Mukha Svanasana.

come to realize that we can breathe into the body in conscious ways, consciously directing the breath to places of tension or holding, and in this come to experience from inside how the breath transforms bodily sensation, emotional feeling, and mental awareness.

Ancient writings on yoga explain this with the *kosha* model, in which prana—the life force that we cultivate through the breath—is the mediating force unifying body and mind (*vayu tattva* in the Samkhya branch of ancient Indian philosophy) (Gambhirananda 1989). Rather than starting from the assumption that the body and mind are somehow separate, here we approach the practice as one of awakening to the existing reality of the bodymind as already whole—wholeness that we might not think or feel to be whole due to the conditions of the bodymind itself in its inner nature and all its sociocultural conditioning.[23] In practicing, when we breathe consciously into a part of the body as directed by the tension highlighted in a particular asana, we are creating the opportunity to consciously awaken awareness there. Doing this in each of 840,000 asanas—the number mentioned in the Hatha Yoga Pradipika as a way of saying there is infinite possibility—we gradually awaken awareness throughout the entirety of our being, awakening and expanding embodied consciousness—even if relatively hidden, dazed, or confused—that is already there.

As a yoga teacher you have the opportunity to guide your students in a way that supports their fullest development of these qualities of awareness. As discussed earlier, many people learn most easily and thereby also open more fully to the transformative potential and effects of yoga and other awakening practices through touch, thus making touch among the resources you might well tap in your teaching. The specific ways that some unique individuals' embodied intelligence manifests in their being may make it practically impossible for them to independently find their way into and out of asanas in a way that is safe, sustainable, and effective, let alone into clearer awareness, often resulting in the reinforcement of postural and life habits that are self-limiting rather than wholesome and transformational. The part of the neuromuscular system that gives us part of our inner self-perception—proprioceptive ("perceiving of self") functions—is often inaccurate, making our larger kinesthetic awareness of movement and positioning in space less than accurate.[24] Clearly informed and appropriately given touch can help students in developing and refining this awareness as they learn to more consciously breathe in their bodymind. Breathing more consciously in the bodymind, perhaps accompanied with the teacher's clear, simple touch, students can awaken to even deeper and clearer self-awareness. In your role as a guide, taking the seat of the teacher, you can give your students support for a lifetime of betterment and joy in their personal practice.

Ethics in Teaching and Touching

The role of the yoga teacher is to provide inspired support and informed guidance to students pursuing their varied and changing aims in doing yoga. When teachers create safe and nurturing yoga classes where students can explore and experience anew in their bodymind, amazing things start to happen. New sensations arise. Breathing consciously becomes a powerful tool of awareness. The bodymind becomes clearer and stronger, emotions even out, the heart opens, and one's sense of spirit soars. One simply feels better—more vibrant, more alive.

Where one goes with this—how one sets and cultivates intention in doing yoga and living their life—can be profoundly affected by the teacher-student relationship. And whatever effects there are will be magnified through touch.[25] Indeed, the physical intimacy of human touch brings ethical and personal considerations to the forefront in giving hands-on guidance and support. Everyone comes to their experience of physical intimacy in unique ways. The same adjustment can feel welcome to one student but invasive to another. What is comfortable for one student might trigger deeply embodied emotional trauma in another. What is welcome with a particular student one day might not be on another day or even in another moment.

The ethical precepts given in the Yoga Sutras of Patanjali are a useful starting place in approaching physical cues, beginning with the intertwined values of *ahimsa*, not hurting, and *satya*, truthfulness. Respecting ahimsa in offering tactile guidance starts with being truthful with yourself about what you know and what you don't know as well as your intention in touching. As with teaching in general, it is important to share and give from a place of

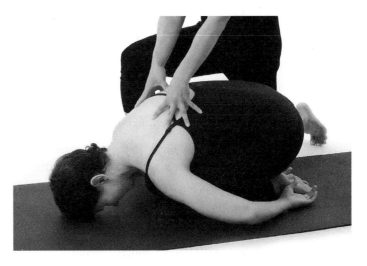

Comforting a student in Balasana (Child's Pose).

truthful understanding, loving kindness, and respect. If you don't understand what's happening with a student in an asana, you are not prepared to give that person a physical cue. By allowing the clarity of your intention in giving physical cues to arise from your knowledge and skill in seeing and relating to students in asanas—including at least a basic understanding of the functional anatomy, risk issues, and contraindications of any asanas you teach—you will be more effective in giving appropriate cues that help your students to deepen their practice.

The intimate quality of touch can also stimulate reactions that bear on matters of *brahmacharya*, the *yama* loosely translated in recent times as "right use of energy" or "moderation" but which originally meant "celibacy"—a perfectly unambiguous term—in the renunciate practices of classical yoga and some contemporary approaches. There is a wide range of views on sex and yoga and on sexual relations between teachers and students. At one extreme is an insistence on celibacy, particularly in renunciate lineages, which might settle the matter (but often doesn't). At the other extreme we find near-complete license given to teachers in acting on sexual attraction to students, as in John Friend's (2006, 92) clearly problematic guidance given in his Anusara teacher-training manual: "When a sexual attraction occurs between you and a student, wait some weeks before acting on the attraction."

As Esther Myers stresses, sexual feelings tend to arise naturally in many students, teachers, or both, leading to or heightening existing feelings of attraction, transference, and projection. Myers (2002, 3) notes that, "While most yoga teachers today are not choosing to be celibate, our ethical practice as teachers requires brahmacharya in relation to our students." When this attitude is embedded in our intention, we're better able to approach any student with clarity expressed through our physical energy that unambiguously conveys compassionate caring free of any confusing, distracting, or otherwise inappropriate thoughts or feelings. Should such thoughts or feelings arise, let that signify that it is time to step away and reexamine your intention and purpose in working closely with your students. Should you perceive such feelings arising in a student, consider creating more distance between you and the student and give only those adjustments that you are confident of being clearly understood by the student as support for their practice and not an expression of personal interest or desire.

These considerations and sensibilities are forms of external guidance generated by what are widely regarded as authoritative texts and underlined in the ethics statements adopted by Yoga Alliance and other professional yoga organizations.

But as Donna Farhi (2006, 18) wisely reminds us, in order for ethical standards to find expression in the reality of relationships, they must operate from an internal locus of ethical being that allows one to properly understand the ethics involved in a specific situation. She offers the example of hugging a student who is grieving and who has asked to be held in contrast to hugging a student who has expressed romantic or sexual interest. When the internal locus is clear and strong, one knows the right

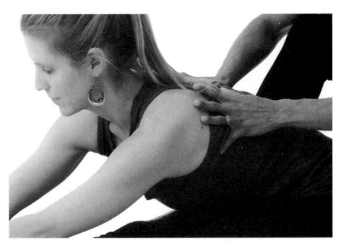

Touch is inherently intimate.

thing to do with reference to external codes, rules, or standards. While the standards are important in creating a community-wide consensus that helps teachers and students alike to better understand and undertake responsible and acceptable interaction, the fact remains that we are far from having such consensus, and in the end internal values will tend to override external rules.

As noted above, we all experience the touch of others in different ways. It is vitally important to appreciate that many students' relationship to touch is deeply conditioned by trauma, and many of these students are doing yoga as one way of healing and living in greater balance and joy. For some students, *any* form of touch can feel uncomfortable, invasive, or traumatic, possibly causing repressed feelings from traumatic experiences to resurface.[26] As we will discuss in the next chapter, this underlines the basic principle that all yoga teachers should always ask permission before touching a student.

As we revisit these and other ethical questions later in this book, it's important to revisit and reflect upon your own experience and practices in giving and receiving touch so long as you are teaching or practicing yoga. Today, as we find more and more yoga teachers applying Hatha yoga to healing interrelated physical and emotional wounds, this takes on growing importance. In the view of some, touch is absolutely vital in the process of healing and transformation, while for others it is a likely cause of pain or trauma. Like the practice of yoga itself, finding and maintaining a balance between giving considerate and appropriate physical guidance and maintaining clear and respectful boundaries is a lifelong process that will evolve just as you evolve in your awareness as a teacher and practitioner.

The Inner Teacher

There is a story of the Buddha shortly after his enlightenment. Walking through the countryside, he approached a small village where the villagers sensed this incredible energy in their midst. Curious, they ventured to the road he was walking along to better see what they sensed. Cautiously approaching the Buddha, one of the villagers asked him, "What are you—a god, a deity?" The Buddha replied, "No." Taken by his luminosity, another asked, "Are you a wizard or a magician?" Again, the Buddha replied, "No." Because he appeared much like a man, one asked, "Are you a man?" And the Buddha again said, "No." "Then what are you?" asked another villager. The Buddha replied: "I am awake."

This brings us back to where we began in this chapter. In doing yoga, we are gradually awakening to a clearer and truer understanding of who we are in our deepest, innermost being. How did the Buddha awaken? By tuning in. It's the same in yoga: the best teacher one will ever have is alive and well inside. Much of the practice is about coming to hear that inner teacher, to listen to and honor the inner teachings. Many spiritual seekers have sought out external teachers as the source of their own enlightenment. A common instruction is to tell the seeker to walk around a sacred mountain. Upon returning less than enlightened and still asking questions, the teacher repeats the instruction and the pupil follows it, again and again. It's not about walking around the mountain but tuning in inside. Eventually one comes to this—or not. Depending on how one teaches yoga, including in giving appropriate and effective hands-on guidance, we are ideally supporting each student in learning to find and honor his or her inner teacher, thereby nurturing the safe and sustainable development of every student in his or her practice.

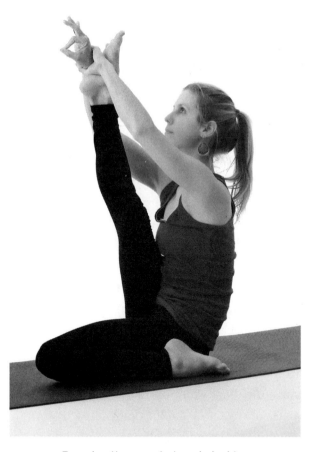

Focusing the gaze to tune in inside.

Chapter 2

The Seven Principles of Hands-On Teaching

CLEAR IN INTENTION AND PURPOSE, STEADY AND CONSISTENT in one's own practice, experienced in and at least generally knowledgeable about yoga, with ongoing study of functional anatomy and basic human pathologies, and an understanding of the interrelated requirements and effects of the asanas one is teaching to inform their sensible sequencing, yoga teachers can offer their students insightful guidance on the yoga practice path. While there is a tendency for some teachers to be random and consequently unclear or confusing in many aspects of teaching yoga due to misunderstanding or a carefree attitude—or, in contrast, to be altogether rigid in applying a universal or predetermined approach to every student or class—we can all learn and refine our repertoire of knowledge and skills, gradually becoming clearer and more effective as we creatively express our experienced and educated sense of how yoga might best be explored and refined as a safe, sustainable, and transformational experience. This is an essential part of the path of the teacher as a yoga guide.

As with the principled rather than random sequencing of asanas that gives us the basic path of a balanced and integrated class, we ideally approach our guidance of asanas in the light of clear principles that inform them, including to whom to offer adjustments, the specific purpose in offering them, what adjustments to give, and when, where, and with what techniques they might best be offered and given. These guiding principles should at least be considered if not honored in keeping with one's larger understanding of yoga, one's philosophy of touch as a medium of support and guidance, as well as one's values and principles in teaching yoga. We will start here with the seven basic principles of hands-on adjustments and how each principle might be best applied in practice.

The Seven Principles of Hands-On Adjustments

Principle 1: Teach What You Know

Principle 2: Ask Permission to Touch

Principle 3: Have Clear Intention

Principle 4: Move with the Breath

Principle 5: Honor Safe Biomechanics

Principle 6: Teach Essential Asana Elements

Principle 7: Support Stable Foundations

Principle 1: Teach What You Know

There is nothing as important in being an authentic and good yoga teacher than teaching what you know and not trying to teach what you don't know. As a principle of hands-on adjustments, teaching what you know involves having a clear understanding of the elements of the asana that can make it safer and more accessible for any given unique student. It is helpful although not necessary to understand variations of the asana that take it farther; however, one should not teach the variations without understanding them.

Teaching what you know starts with getting to know the asanas through years of practice, informed training, and in-depth study. Just because one can do something does not mean he or she fundamentally understands it or can guide others in it; many physically gifted yoga students can do practically any asana, yet this ability does not automatically confer the depth of understanding that transfers into clearly and insightfully guiding others who are exploring it. Indeed, teachers for whom certain asanas have come easily in their personal practice typically have greater difficulty grasping the challenges that others with different physical abilities have in exploring those same asanas. Consequently, the more naturally physically adept teacher is often at a loss in guiding more physically challenged students in doing what that teacher finds simple and straightforward. Meanwhile, less physically adept teachers who have spent years exploring and developing the ability to do certain asanas typically learn more about them and are thus better prepared to offer helpful insights to all of their students.

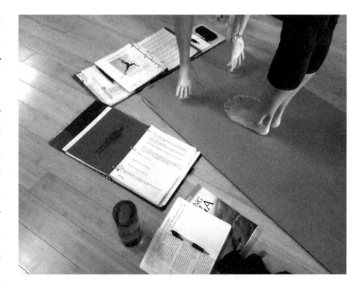

Ongoing practice and study are essential in being a competent teacher.

Applying this principle in practice, we should teach within the limitations of our experience, knowledge, and skills. This helps to ensure that as teachers, we are honoring both our students and ourselves. Acknowledging what we know and what we don't know is also empowering as we accept ourselves for who we are as teachers in the present moment. This acknowledgement reinforces that part of the path of the teacher that is an unending learning journey, opening us to seeing more clearly what we have to offer and how we might further develop in every aspect of our teaching.

There are a variety of ways to learn more about asanas and how to teach them to others. The first step is to maintain a consistent practice and use your own experience on your yoga mat to develop insight. While this is the foundation of all that follows, it is important to bear in mind that what you experience on your mat is just that; others will have different experiences on their mats (or in a chair, or wherever else they might be practicing). You will gain further insight by practicing under a variety of conditions, such as when you are fatigued, anxious, cold, or injured as well as at different times of the day, in different settings, and throughout the seasons—including from young to old across the seasons of one's life. You will go even further in developing your skills and knowledge through in-depth yoga studies, your initial teacher training, and continuing education throughout the life span of your teaching.

At the very minimum you should learn the basic elements of the asanas that you are teaching—their benefits, risks, contraindications, preparatory asanas, alignment principles, energetic actions, common challenges with the asanas, modifications, use of props, and integrative counterposes. This in turn involves studying and learning the fundamentals of yoga anatomy and biomechanics along with common pathologies that are present among at least some students in nearly any class—and having either the insight to intelligently and supportively guide these students or the openness to let them know that you don't have that insight.[1] It's also important to have extensive guidance and practice in learning how to see, understand, and relate in meaningful ways to the diverse array of students likely to be in your classes. Yoga teacher Pattabhi Jois's popular saying, "Practice, and all is coming," is thus both the starting point and the thread that ideally runs through the years of your deepening experience in teaching yoga, even while ideally more deeply studying all that's involved in the practice than suggested by Jois's formula of ninety-nine percent practice, one percent study.

In the next chapter we will look closely at specific hands-on techniques. All of the techniques given should be practiced extensively prior to using them in your teaching. Ideally, you will practice giving hands-on cues under the direct guidance of an experienced mentor teacher as part of your training and continuing education before offering tactile guidance to students in a class. That practice will help you to learn to feel how different students respond to your tactile cues under varying conditions relating to emotion, holding, interaction, gravity, resistance, and positioning. Gaining considerable experience and finding comfort and confidence with hands-on assistance will help you as you explore using other parts of your body to support and guide students. As you gain more experience and expertise, you can explore working with different modalities and making different kinds of adjustments that go beyond the basics, all the while teaching what you know and not what you don't know.

Principle 2: Ask Permission to Touch

For hundreds of years, gurus have touched their disciples with a sense of complete license while at least ostensibly governed by an internal locus of ethical action and informed by an accurate understanding of the student's true needs—indeed, usually considered more accurate than the student's perception. During years of practicing Mysore-style Ashtanga Vinyasa and Iyengar yoga, I became accustomed to teachers using their hands, feet, knees, chest, elbows, and backs to push, pull, and otherwise manipulate my body into preconceived and ostensibly "correct" postural forms with nary a nod to asking permission or querying me about how their adjustments felt. Submission was—and problematically is—in the yoga culture: we watched videos showing our teachers' teachers—always referred to as *guruji*—doing the same to them, often with extremely aggressive technique (such as forcefully lifting the chin to push the crown of the head into the soles of the feet while pushing the feet toward the head in advanced back bends, thereby forcefully hyperextending the cervical spine). In many teacher-training programs, students are told not to question the methods of the trainers and are never given an example of a trainer asking permission before giving hands-on assistance or guidance in the training.

There are several reasons to always ask permission to touch. First, honoring personal boundaries is a matter of basic respect for other people. You can show respect to your students by simply asking, "May I give you hands-on guidance?" or "May I touch you?" While at first it might seem awkward to ask permission before touching, the more one does it, the more natural it feels, to the point that you will feel something is missing when not asking permission.

Second, there is the intimate nature of touch and the fact that different people come to matters of touch in different ways, some welcoming it (sometimes or all the time) and others not (usually or always). The experience of touch varies across the vast landscapes of different cultures, religions, and personal histories.[2] You may not know the cultural, religious, and personal values, sensibilities, or sensitivities of every student in your class. You may have students for whom any touch by some-one of the opposite sex who is not their spouse could violate their religious beliefs. You are likely to have students who have experienced physical trauma that tends to resurface when touched—especially without first giving explicit permission—and who may or may not be a willing or welcoming participant in this form of teacher-student interaction. You might have students who are experiencing and perhaps struggling with transference or projection issues with you, want to be in your class, yet with some degree of confusion may need your active support in maintaining clearer and more comfortable boundaries in your mutual interaction.

Third, people change. You might have a regular student who always welcomes your hands-on support. But in any given moment, you do not necessarily know what's happening with him or her. One's moods can shift, including during a practice, in one moment feeling open to physical contact, and a few moments later feeling like being left alone. Our physical condition changes as well, whether during a practice or from something that has happened off the mat. You might have a regular student who slightly sprained her ankle; she absolutely does not need you to emphasize rooting that foot as she ordinarily would in Trikonasana (Triangle Pose).

The simplest way to ask permission to touch is to ask permission to touch. That is not a typo. You can play with many variations to the question: "May I give you hands-on guidance?" "Is it okay for me to press here so you can better understand what I'm trying to say?" "Is it okay for me to give you adjustments with my hands?" With students you've come to know well and who are always open to your tactile guidance, you might find mutual comfort in initially and lightly placing your hands on them in a way they've experienced with you many times before and simply ask, "Is this okay?" True to your ethical ways, in your integrity as a teacher and honoring the integrity of your students, you will find a way to share in this quality of communication with your students in a way that feels natural to you and naturally and unambiguously clear to them.

There are some methods of asking permission that are not recommended. First, do not ask for a show of hands to indicate who does or does not want hands-on support. This creates peer pressure. Some students will not feel comfortable raising a hand, and some might change how they feel later in class—plus you might forget who said yes or no. Second, do not rely on students giving blanket permission when completing an initial new student registration form; again, conditions—and people—change. Third, using cards that are red on one side and green on the other and asking students to turn the card to indicate their preference not only takes students out of their practice, it assumes they remember what it indicates and that they still feel that way. Simply always ask permission to touch.

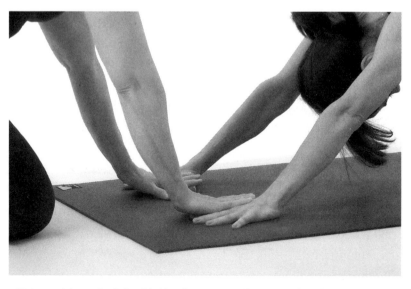

Giving guidance in Adho Mukha Svanasana (Downward-Facing Dog Pose).

As you are giving an adjustment, check in with the student by asking, "Is this okay?" This is important because the student might change his or her mind about the contact once it's happening. Again, when working with students with whom you are very familiar and have a good understanding of their practice, those with whom you might, through mutual and explicit assent, discover that it is generally okay to touch and whom you've asked "Is this okay" as you are beginning to make contact, check in during the physical cueing for reaffirmation that whatever you are doing is still okay.

Principle 3: Have Clear Intention

Before approaching a student to ask permission to give hands-on guidance, be as clear as you can in your intention. Drawing from what you know and what you see in that moment, consider how you can use individualized verbal cues and further demonstration to achieve an effect prior to offering tactile assistance or adjustment. Give the student the opportunity to respond to your words and modeling before offering to use your hands. Drawing further from your knowledge and observation of the student, know what you want to do before doing it while remaining attuned to your student and open to changing what you're doing based on that listening. Once given permission by the student, explain what you are encouraging and doing as you begin to touch the student.

Appreciating that students' bodies will respond in different ways, be as clear and specific as you can in giving the cue or adjustment without attachment to a specific preconceived outcome—even as you have clarity in your intention. Go with their response in refining your interaction with them. Feel, communicate, and adapt as you go. *Aparigraha,* the yama meaning "not grasping" in doing yoga, applies equally to your intention in giving assistance and to guiding your students in letting the asana most naturally come to them without forcing it. Sometimes teachers become attached to a certain preconception of what a student can or should be able to do in refining or deepening an asana rather than staying attuned to observing how the asana seems to be presenting itself to the student and evolving in each wave of breath. This can result in pushing students too far, taking them out of their practice, and undermining their sense of trust in opening to inner awareness and guidance.

Similarly, students are often attached to their own idea of how or how far to go and may ask for a more intense adjustment than you think their body is ready for at that moment. Navigating these tendencies depends on staying with your larger intention and purpose as a teacher and encouraging your students to stay with the asana practice as a source of deepening self-awareness and self-transformation in which the "less is more" adage has much currency. In a world in which most people all too often feel judged, yoga classes should offer a space where students can feel fully accepted for who they are, intrinsically beautiful and perfect in that moment. Yet as teachers, we carry a responsibility for honestly conveying to students our sincere best insights into what they are doing in their practice and how it might be refined, made simpler, and taken deeper. This inevitably includes seeing value in the student doing something different from what he or she might presently be doing and then conveying that insight through our words and other actions.

For example, if a student's front knee is splayed inward and projects out beyond her heel in Utthita Parsvakonasana (Extended Side Angle Pose), you will see and appreciate the benefit of realigning her knee to be centered above her heel as a means of protecting her anterior cruciate and medial collateral ligaments (and the patella tendon as well as related structural effects in the hip, pelvis, and spine). Rather than communicating this as a "correction," try to find language and qualities of voice that convey the beauty of what she's doing in harmony with the support you're offering in suggesting and even physically cueing the realignment. For example, you might say, "Good; keep rooting down into your feet, and see how it feels to bring your foot farther forward to align your knee just above your heel, which is a more stable position and better for your knee." You might give a light tactile cue encouraging her to press her knee slightly out, aligning it toward the center of her foot, and simply add, "Beautiful. Stay with the breath." (Yes, saying "beautiful" is judgmental, and a case can be made for never saying anything that is judgmental; still, I'll go with sparingly giving such affirmative judgments.)

Whether working with new or experienced students, consider giving them the space to explore asanas free of your individualized attention. New students can feel overwhelmed by the newness of basic postures, by *ujjayi pranayama* and all the many nuances of the practice—aligning, gazing, breathing, transitioning, feeling inside for ultimate guidance, and so much more. Often the best approach with new students is to leave them largely on their own unless you see them doing something that could cause an injury, giving them the opportunity to experience what it's like to be in your class and in their bodymind in a new way. Let this be part of your intention. As students gain more experience and you give them more individual guidance, occasionally give them periods of several classes or even weeks where you attentively observe them from a distance, giving them the space to explore more on their own. Be equally clear when working with more experienced students to be just as attentive to how their body is responding, and resist giving strong, aggressive adjustments—even when asked. Stay with your intention.

Principle 4: Move with the Breath

Conscious breathing in the asana practice is what most distinguishes yoga from most other expressions of bodymind and physical practice culture. It is what most gives yoga its transformative potential and opens the windows of perception to clearer awareness and a more balanced, awakened life. In doing yoga, we ideally breathe with our awareness in the breath and use this awareness to direct the breath as suggested by the sensations arising is the asana. Going with this sensibility, in teaching yoga we ideally cue students with the preface of "Inhaling . . . ," "Exhaling . . . ," "Staying with the breath . . . ," or other ways of verbalizing the connection of breath to movement and to energetic actions within and between the asanas. The words *inhaling* and *exhaling* are ideally followed by a related verbal cue to do something rather than saying "inhale, exhale." For example, in guiding the transition from Tadasana (Mountain Pose) to Urdhva Hastasana (Upward Hands Pose) to Uttanasana (Standing Forward Bend Pose), one might cue as follows: "Exhaling completely, turn your palms out. With your inhalation, slowly extend your arms out and up overhead; exhaling, slowly swan-dive forward and down to Uttanasana."

In hands-on teaching and in other ways of working closely with an individual student, it is important to tune in to the student's breathing. Observation of the student's breathing provides you with keener insight into what is happening with the student in his or her practice. As a barometer of the practice, the breath reflects a number of qualities. Is the student breathing deeply and smoothly? Is there an ujjayi quality to the breath? Are there natural pauses between inhalations and exhalations? If you are not getting a sense of "yes" to each of these questions, it is likely that the student is either not present in the practice, is straining, or both. In any case, ask your student to come back into the breath, which may require that he or she back off from the asana or modify it in ways that allow the breath to flow more steadily and easily—again, encouraging an abiding sense of the asanas finding expression around and through the integrity of the breath rather than trying to squeeze the breath into asanas and transitional movements.

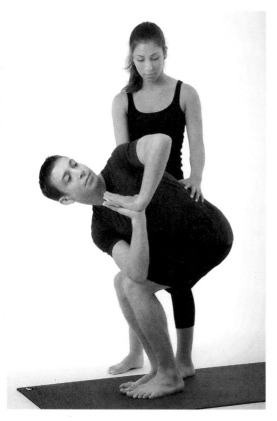

Synchronize your breathing with your student's breathing.

In giving hands-on guidance, we ideally breathe with the student and synchronize our physical cues with the student's breath. After detecting the student's breathing pattern or asking the student to breathe deeply, synchronize your own breathing with your student's breathing. This will help ensure that your cues go with the student's breath. Whether or not you're continuing to verbally cue the connection of breath and action, your hands will now be guiding the student to refine their positioning or energetic actions with the natural support arising in the phases of the breath.

For example, in working with a student in Paschimottanasana (West Stretching Pose or Seated Forward Fold), you might have one or both hands initially pressing down on the pelvis to emphasize the steady rooting of the sitting bones, which is the primary energetic action of all seated forward folds, hip openers, and twists. Meanwhile, you want to encourage maximum lengthening of the spine and continued opening across the heart center, which is well facilitated by the student slightly lifting the torso up on each inhalation and then, lifting the sternum, moving farther forward and perhaps down on the exhalations. With your hands on the student, watching and feeling for the rhythm of the student's breath, you should coordinate your breathing with his or hers as you give tactile cues that accentuate the verbal cues to move in this wavelike fashion in connection with the breath, breath by breath releasing slightly more deeply into the asana with an elongated spine.

There is another valuable aspect of teaching with the breath: your own presence of mind and attentiveness to your student. By taking in a deep breath that connects your own breathing to your student's breathing patterns, you will naturally come into more awareness of what is happening in that moment with you, your student, and the rest of the class. In this practice, both you as the teacher and your student in his or her practice will more fully sense clearer inner awakening as conscious breathing creates a deeper opening to the wholeness of bodymind.

Principle 5: Honor Safe Biomechanics

There are certain ways that the body most easily and stably moves or is held in position. There are also ways it can move or be held that cause pain, instability, or injury. For example, if standing in Tadasana, one fully internally rotates the arms and attempts to reach them out and up overhead, the top of the arm bones (the humeral heads) will jam up against the ends of the shoulders (the acromion processes) in the vast preponderance of students. By first externally rotating the arms, it creates the necessary space in the joints for the arms to rise overhead free of this impingement. Similarly, in Sirsasana I (Headstand) it is vitally important to position the top of the head on the floor and maintain the neutral extension of the cervical spine; placement of the head in any other way can injure the neck.

In working with students, it is important to understand and honor the ideal biomechanical functioning of the body. This starts, again, with practice, study, and training, but in practical application relies on the teacher's commitment to bringing this understanding into the practice of guiding students in their asana practices. There are several specific aspects of biomechanics that are of utmost importance.

First, when guiding students into safely aligned positioning, always first cue and encourage active joint movement—conscious, voluntary movement created by the student through muscular action—so that they are creating the locomotion

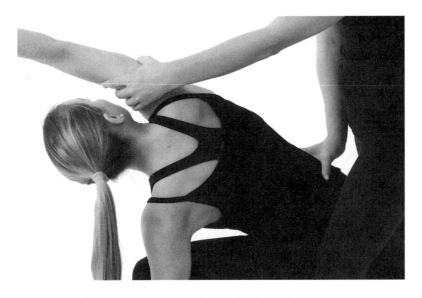

Giving a proximal cue in Utthita Parsvakonasana.

and feeling its effects before considering or offering to provide passive joint movement (hands-on adjustments). Put differently, do your best to stay out of the way, allowing your students to be in their practice as autonomously as can be, exploring and learning from the inside how to find stability and ease along with your visual and verbal cues, and only then and with permission offer tactile guidance.[3] (As we explore in chapter 3, passive joint movement is just one type of tactile cue, while many others do not involve locomotion).

Second, work as proximally—nearest the midline—as appropriate in adjusting a student in an asana, and give only very light suggestive cues when the touch is fully distal. Phrased another way, never give a strong tactile cue distally, such as turning the hand to create external rotation or any other repositioning of the arm in Utthita Parsvakonasana, which can dislocate the arm of a student with hypermobile shoulder joints. When working distally, you have greater mechanical advantage and can inadvertently cause injury.[4] A few additional examples to further clarify this point:

- Pulling back on the shoulders in back bends such as Urdhva Mukha Svanasana (Upward-Facing Dog Pose) or Bhujangasana (Cobra Pose). This adjustment is distal to the lumbar spine segment, causing excessive and possibly injurious pressure to the lower back. If you think a student can benefit from pulling his or her shoulders back, cue this verbally, with demonstration, or with a very light suggestive touch while emphasizing the roots and energetic actions of the asana in the feet, legs, and pelvis along with spaciousness up the spine and across the chest.

- Pulling back on the hand in Parivrtta Trikonasana (Revolved Triangle Pose). This adjustment is distal to the shoulder and can cause overstretching or excessive range of motion in the glenohumeral joint, which is especially problematic for students with instability or impingement in or around the rotator cuff; the leveraged mechanical advantage one has in such an adjustment is also distal to the lumbar spine and can cause excessive rotation there.

- Lifting up on the elevated heel in Utthita Hasta Padangusthasana (Extended Hand to Big Toe Pose). This is distal to the tendinous origins of the hamstring muscles at the ischial tuberosities (the sitting bones) and can cause excessive stretching at this place that is most vulnerable to hamstring strain as well as in the bodies and insertion points of the hamstring muscles.

Third, do not apply direct pressure on vulnerable joints, organs, or injured areas. Rather, find the natural "handles" on the body in any given pose (all of which are shown in part II). In giving adjustments in or near joints, begin with your understanding of that joint, including the type of joint, its movements, and its safe range of motion. There is only very rarely any value in placing your hands on a student's abdomen or elsewhere that is close to internal organs. In doing so, the cues should be light, specific, and suggestive, never strong, general, or locomotive. Do not press into the organs. (Remember, you are teaching yoga, not giving a massage!) Be particularly aware of student injuries—of all sorts—and listen very closely to what your student is expressing about it before considering any form of touch.

Fourth, feel and watch for how the student's body is responding to your verbal and tactile cues, including shifts in other parts of his or her body and signs of increased tension. It is important to appreciate that in giving attention to one part of an asana, there is typically less attention elsewhere. When refining alignment, energetic actions, or otherwise doing something different in one part of an asana, there is a tendency for whatever is no longer in one's primary attention to change. For instance, when cueing stronger action in the back leg in Virabhadrasana II (Warrior II Pose), the tendency is for the knee in the front leg to splay in and the front hip to splay out. When cueing further rotation of the torso in Parivrtta Parsvakonasana (Revolved Extended Side Angle Pose), the back foot tends to lose its equal rooting, the front hip tends to shift out, and that knee tends to splay in. With practice and experience you will learn to anticipate these unintended consequences of your focused guidance, and you will incorporate this larger set of considerations into the cue that you are most focused on with your student in that moment.

Fifth, if in your observation there are fundamental misalignments or other sources of instability or potential strain, consider asking the student to come partially or completely out of the asana. Be patient, explain your concerns, and then reguide the student into the asana while further addressing the issues that led you to ask him or her to come out of it. If this observation is made close to when you will cue the class to transition to the other side of the same asana, try to work directly with that student in setting up and transitioning into it on the second side so that the rhythm of the class is maintained.

Principle 6: Teach Essential Asana Elements

In teaching asanas, we are ideally creating space and offering guidance that helps students to develop a sense of both the whole of the practice as well as the elements that give the asanas their sustainable and transformational potential. In doing so, it is important to give physical cues in a way that clearly conveys the essential elements of each asana, as follows:

- **stability and ease:** Nearly every asana has a slightly different foundation that creates unique opportunities for students to explore and learn grounding actions. To the extent that one is continuously rooting down to create a more stable foundation, space is created in the joints, and with it, greater overall ease. Without conscious grounding, the tendency is to lose stability and ease or to create unnecessary tension. For example, a common tendency in doing Paschimottanasana is to focus so intently on the forward folding movement that one loses the steady rooting of their sitting bones, which is the primary energetic action for grounding and initiating all seated forward folds, twists, and hip openers. This causes compression—and potentially strain—in the lumbar spine and compromises the fuller elongation of the spine, expansiveness of the heart center, and fullness of the breath. More generally and importantly, in giving cues, first give your attention to what might be most at risk—which may involve the use of props or other modifications—and then focus on establishing the firm and relaxed foundation of the asana through specific grounding pressure that is informed by the alignment principles and larger energetic actions of the particular asana. There are similarly important grounding actions in every family of asanas that should be given attention early in the cueing process. Again, note how, in giving attention to one aspect of an asana, there is a tendency for other aspects of it to fade from awareness and thus fade from one's effort, especially the stabilizing and easing foundation of the asana. Thus, when giving any physical cue, stay attuned to the effects of that cue on the basic foundation of the asana.

- **alignment principles:** The functional anatomy and biomechanics of each asana gives us its alignment principles, which tell us how best to position the body in each asana.[5] When the alignment principles of any given asana are embodied in the practice, students find easier access to stability and ease while further ensuring the maximum benefits of their practice. When one misunderstands or ignores basic alignment principles, the benefits of the asana can largely be lost while its risks are increased. It is thus vitally important to give demonstrations along with succinct and clear verbal instructions when guiding students into an asana. It is equally important to adapt basic alignment principles to the unique conditions of different students rather than insisting on one way for everybody—adaptations that should be offered only when informed by an understanding of the student's condition and the elements and effects of the modified position. These methods of instruction can then be enhanced with hands-on cues that guide students into safe and sustainable positions, including with the use of props and other modifications.

- **energetic actions:** As discussed above, it is important first to establish the foundation of each asana. From the foundation that one creates through grounding actions and alignment, it is easier then to create other energetic actions that help to refine the integrity of the overall asana. The concept of energetic actions expands on the idea of lines of energy. Energetic actions start with running lines of energy to enhance grounding and to help create opening, then from this foundation moves into extension, flexion, rotation, lateral flexion, contraction, and expansion, all of which can be highlighted with specific hands-on cues. For example, in Bakasana (Crane Pose, often erroneously translated as "Crow Pose," which is Kakasana), the fingers are spread wide apart (the thumbs not so wide as to overstretch the ligaments and place undue pressure on the nerves in the thenar space between the index finger and the thumb), and there is ideally equal pressure across the entire span of each hand as well as out and down through the fingers and thumbs. Meanwhile, one wants to work from this foundation to more fully root the shoulder blades down against the back ribs, fully extend the elbows, squeeze the knees against the outer shoulders (enhanced by the energetic action of *pada bandha* in the feet as the heels and sides of the balls of the feet are pressed together), elevate the heels toward the buttocks, lightly engage the abdominal core, and thereby elevate the pelvis higher. In Utthita Parsvakonasana, we run a strong line of energy down the back leg and foot to root down while stretching from that rooted foot out through the arm that is stretched overhead. To this we add several energetic actions: pada bandha in the feet, isometric outward spiraling of the front foot to foster alignment of the front knee, thigh, and hip, extension of the back leg, rotation of the torso, external rotation of the upper arm, lengthening of the lower side of the torso, a line of energy from the lower shoulder into the hand and the floor, and expansion of the heart center, all of which can be given with subtle hands-on cues—and all of which lend to the stability, ease, sustainability, refinement, and deepening of the effects of this asana.

- **transitioning in, refining,** and **transitioning out:** How we approach an asana shapes how we experience it and how we can refine it, which in turn influences the experience of coming out of the asana with stability and ease. In transitioning in, it is important first to establish the initial foundation with the proper alignment of whatever will be the source of grounding along with energetic actions that enhance this foundation and facilitate stable, safe, and comfortable transitional movement. Once in the asana, we apply the breath and energetic actions to refine and deepen our exploration and expression of it. We then apply specific energetic actions to more simply and easily transition out. For example, strongly rooting down through the legs and feet in preparation for Utthita Trikonasana (Extended Triangle Pose) awakens the leg muscles and creates the foundation from which to lengthen the torso out over the front leg. Once there, the slight energetic action of spiraling the front foot outward (without it actually moving) helps press the hip of that leg under toward the other hip, which in combination with pressing the back leg more strongly in extension makes this asana more of a hip opener. In preparing to come out of the asana, if one runs a strong line of energy from the hip to the heel of the back leg, this will make it easier on the lower back in bringing the torso back upright. Hands-on cues should highlight each of these stages of practice and guidance, not just what is happening in the asana qua asana.

Principle 7: Support Stable Foundations

The physical starting point in giving all hands-on assistance and guidance is the cultivation of a stable foundation, starting with your physical foundation as a teacher. If you are not stable in your own foundation, you will compromise the support you might otherwise be giving to your students while possibly setting yourself up for injury. Taking at least a breath to position yourself stably, comfortably, and appropriately for giving what support you might be offering, you will be in a better position to give that support and continue giving support throughout your lifetime as a teacher.

Having established your own foundation and after giving primary attention to whatever might be most at risk to the student in the asana, turn your attention and cueing to the student's foundation in the asana—or in transitioning in or out of it as the case may be. If the foundation is not properly established, something else about the asana or transition will be compromised. Thus, aside from immediately addressing primary risks, it makes no sense whatsoever to focus initially on something other than the foundation of the asana when teaching it; to do so can further undermine the foundation and unnecessarily create problems. For example, we commonly find ill-informed instruction in which a teacher is showing how to guide a student into better alignment in Parivrtta Trikonasana by first focusing on how to reposition the torso, spine, shoulders, and arms—even giving instruction to let off the foundation in the feet and legs in order to arrive at what the teacher considers better alignment in those parts of the upper body, thereby undermining the very foundation upon which the asana is built. The foundation-first approach starts with the positioning and actions in the feet, legs, hips, and pelvis from the ground up, and then develops the asana farther up the body with whatever modifications and use

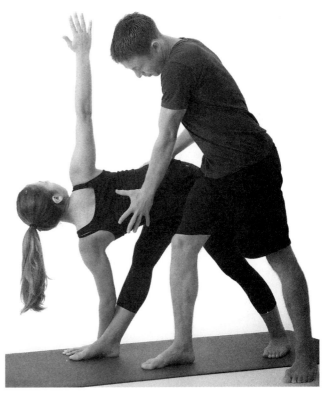

Always give yourself a stable foundation for supporting your students.

of props might best support the student going further into stability, ease, and openness without ever changing the foundation of the asana. If it appears (and more importantly, feels to the student) that the problem is in the foundation itself, then start over with modification of the foundation, perhaps with props, so that the foundation is stable, and proceed from there. With your own ego safely checked at the door, you will be more interested in guiding your students in how they go— starting and continuing with stability and ease—than in how far they go, especially since compromising the foundation compromises everything else.

The principles presented here represent a synthesis of shared, practice-based insight, study, training, and years of teaching and training teachers in diverse settings. Yet in the end, they are only principles, while in teaching yoga we are human beings interacting with other human beings, ideally even more deeply guided by the core values we bring to our practice and our service than the principles that might give us guidance in our words and actions. Starting with and remaining true to your core values will make the principles offered here and that you find elsewhere in the vast universe of yoga resources more meaningful and useful in the practical sharing of your knowledge and skills as a yoga teacher. With your values and principles alive in the intelligence and spirit of your bodymind, the specific ways you show up with your students in guiding their practices will naturally evolve to be the best they can be.

Chapter 3

Foundations and Techniques in Giving Yoga Adjustments

GIVING EFFECTIVE HANDS-ON GUIDANCE STARTS WITH the preparation that allows you to most easily translate the concepts, sensitivities, and principles discussed in the previous chapters to the practical realities of working with individual students. This preparation includes learning specific techniques for using your hands and other parts of your body, techniques that are covered in detail in this chapter and applied to specific asanas in part II. The first step in this preparation involves stepping back to consider several important factors that will largely determine what to do or not do in giving physical cues.

First and foremost, it is important to have at least some modicum of clarity about the student before giving guidance (verbal or nonverbal). Put differently, the art and science of touching in giving hands-on adjustments begins with seeing—and understanding what you are seeing. This starts with a conversation with the student about any injuries or other conditions that might be significant in his or her asana practice or in receiving hands-on support. Ideally, you have this conversation before class starts and from time to time thereafter as long as the student comes to your classes. It is important to ask specifically about any recent or chronic pain, strain or sprain, recent or chronic illness, current or recent pregnancy, or any other conditions that might be a factor in the asana or pranayama practices—in whatever you are teaching. Check in from time to time with regular ongoing students to see how they are doing and if anything significant has changed since you last checked in. With both new and ongoing students, try to tune in to body language, facial expression, and breathing patterns to further assess their condition.

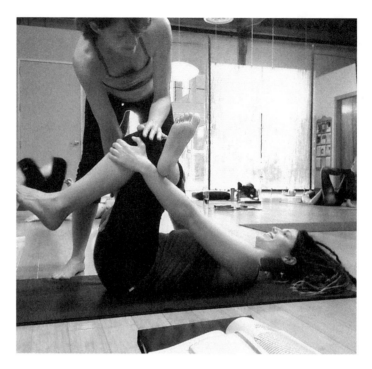

Establish clear and open communication with all students.

In introducing yourself to a new student, try to ask the questions listed to inform your assessment of the student and how best to guide him or her in their practice.

Initial Student Query

1. *Have you ever practiced yoga? If so, what style, for what period of time, and how frequently?*

2. *Do you have any injuries or anything else going on with your body that I should be aware of? How are your ankles, knees, hips, back, shoulders, neck, and wrists?*

3. If a student reports having an injury or issue, follow up with more specific questions: *What is it about your knee? Have you had surgery? When? How does it feel now?* Based on the answers to these questions, give the student some initial guidance on how he or she might modify his or her practice. Use your knowledge but also be prepared to acknowledge that you do not know about the injury or issue, and encourage the student to take care of him- or herself.

4. *Are you pregnant, or have you recently had a baby?* Ask this of any woman you think might be in childbearing years and then share with her the basic trimester cautions described in chapter 11 of *Teaching Yoga* and the sequencing given for different conditions and stages of pregnancy in chapter 8 of *Yoga Sequencing*.

5. *What is your work or daily life like?* This question can provide insight into chronic stress, pain, tightness, and weakness as well as larger lifestyle conditions that might affect one's practice.

6. *What do you do for exercise?* This can tell you a lot about chronic tightness or pain. If the student answers that he or she does not exercise, this is also important information.

Learning to See and Understand Students in Asanas

Self-reporting is not a guarantee that you will get accurate or complete information on a student's condition; many people are reluctant to share personal information with relative strangers, are unaware of a condition, or are in denial about the significance of some conditions. Your ability to accurately see and better understand students in asanas starts with learning to see bodies more generally, specifically learning to see and understand different bodies from various perspectives. This essential skill is best developed through anatomical and asana observation clinics in yoga teacher workshops, including the basic methods of partner standing observation, asana laboratory observation, and practice teaching observation, the insights from which you will further develop in apprenticing with a mentor teacher and ideally for as long as you are teaching yoga. This observational skill development is best done in conjunction with learning the fundamentals of functional anatomy in the context of yoga teacher training.

Step 1: Partner Standing Observation

Partner up with another teacher or trainee, one in the role as the "looker" and the other as the "lookee." The looker uses a worksheet with three illustrations of the body in anatomical position (front, back, and side) to record their observations. There is no judgment about any of the findings. The lookees take a few marching steps forward and then stop and stand in a normal position as if waiting in line for a movie. They will be in this position for a few minutes. Ask them not to try to change or correct their posture as the looker observes and records. Ideally the lookee's clothes allow his or her posture to be easily observed from foot to head. With the looker squatting behind their partner, the observation begins at the feet:

- **feet:** Are the feet straight? One foot out, one foot in? Flat-footed or high-arched?
- **Achilles:** Do they align straight, veer toward the midline or toward the lateral?
- **calves:** Look and feel. Is there more tension in one calf than the other? Is there more tension on the outside or the inside of the calf?
- **knees:** Is the back of the knee hard or soft, flexed, extended, or hyperextended?
- **hips:** Place the palms flat on the hips facing downward with thumbs straight across the sacrum. Are the hips level?
- **arms:** Do they hang evenly at the side, or is one hand more in front than the other? Where are the palms facing? Is there a carrying angle at the elbow?
- **shoulders:** Are they even or level? Does one shoulder ride higher than the other?
- **head:** Is it centered between the shoulders? Does the head tilt or rotate to the side?

Now the looker stands perpendicularly to the side of their partner and observes the following:

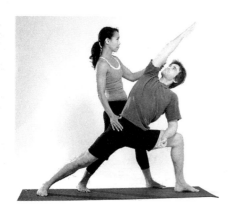

Practice learning to see postural tendencies.

- Does the ear hole (external auditory meatus) line up over the shoulder? Does the head move forward or behind the shoulder? Are the shoulders either slumping forward or pulled back?
- Does the shoulder line up over the hip?
- Is the upper back hunched (kyphosis)? Is the chest collapsed?
- Does the hip line up over the knee? Is the pelvis pitched either forward or back?
- Does the knee line up over the ankle? Is it hyperextended?
- Does the ear hole line up over the ankle?

Now the looker stands in front of their partner and observes the following:

- What do you notice about that person's feet? Are they noticeably different from this view?

- Do the kneecaps point forward? Do the knees collapse to the midline, are they straight, or do they bow to the side?

- Do the hips show rotation? How about the torso—any rotation there?

- Is one arm more anterior than the other? Where do the hands fall by the sides?

- Are the shoulders still at the same level?

- How about the person's head? What do you notice from this position?

Now take about five minutes to share the findings with the lookee, without judgment, and then switch roles. If done as part of a group process, come together and ask, "Who has perfect posture?" You will only very rarely find anyone free of some postural anomaly.

Step 2: Asana Laboratory Observation

The yoga teacher-training asana laboratory is one of the most effective methods for learning to look at, see, and relate to students in the asana practice. Preparation for this exercise includes prior reading about the asana under focus, study of its basic functional anatomy, alignment principles and energetic actions, plus experience practicing the asana under different conditions (time of day, time of year, moods, qualities of well-being, and so on). The basic method is to look separately at each of three or four "model" students—usually co-participants in a teacher-training program or continuing-education workshop—whose varied expressions of the selected asana display the different challenges typically found in a class of students: tightness, weakness, hypermobility, instability, misalignment, and so on. Proceed as follows; here we use the example of Parivrtta Trikonasana (Revolved Triangle Pose):

- Before asking someone to model an asana, encourage him or her to honor their own needs for safety and comfort, including the option to modify or come out of the asana whenever they wish. Encourage everyone else in the group to offer questions and insights in a sensitive yet honest manner.

- Ask the model participant to come into the asana based on their sense of how to do so. Do not give any initial verbal cues, allowing her to guide herself into the asana. Encourage her to switch sides whenever she feels the

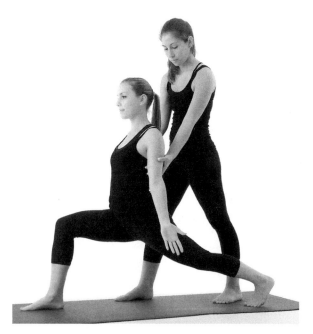

Get off your mat to see your students more clearly.

need while trying to stay in it on each side as long as she comfortably can. If she modifies the positioning that you are expecting her to display (for example, a hyperextended knee), cue her to move into that tendency to the extent that she feels comfortable so that the observers can see that tendency.

- Take about a minute to observe the student, walking 360 degrees around her. Remember that asanas are an expression of unique human beings, not an ideal or static form or "pose."

- Bring your observation first to whatever is most at risk in the asana. While asking yourself what is happening there, ask the model participant how she feels in that part of her body.

Now look more comprehensively at the model student's entire expression of the asana:

- **breath and general vibe:** How is she breathing? Does she look comfortable? Anxious? Balanced? Steady? Comfortable?

- **feet and ankles:** How are they aligned? Is the front foot turned out ninety degrees? Does it appear that the feet are rooting and awakening with pada bandha? Where does the weight appear to be—inner foot, outer foot, balanced? Are the toes softly rooting or clenching? What is happening with the arches?

- **knees:** Is the kneecap aligned toward the center of the front foot? Is the knee bent into flexion or hyperextension? Is the kneecap revealing activation of the quadriceps?

- **pelvis:** Is it level and even, pitched forward in anterior rotation, back in posterior rotation, or close to neutral? Does she appear to be drawing the sitting bone of the front leg back and down as if toward the heel of the back foot?

- **spine:** What is its position in the lumbar area as it extends from the pelvis? Is there an extreme lateral bend or twisting? Does there appear to be any compression in the spine? What curves do you see going up into the thoracic and cervical sections of the spine?

- **rib cage:** Are the lower front ribs protruding out or softening in? Are the back ribs rounded? Are the upper side ribs protruding? What do these observations tell you about the spine?

- **chest and collarbones:** Is the torso aligned straight out over the front leg, or is it leaning forward? Is the torso revolving open, lateral to the floor, or turned toward the floor? Is the chest expansive? Are the collarbones spreading away from each other?

- **shoulders, arms, hands, and fingers:** Are the shoulder blades drawing down against the back ribs, or tending to draw up toward the ears? Is the lower shoulder rolled forward or drawn back and down? Are the arms reaching out away from each other perpendicular to the floor? Are they fully extended? Are the elbows straight, bent, or hyperextended? Are the palms fully open and the fingers fully extended?

- **Where is the student's energy?** Where does it appear she is applying herself with effort? Rooting down strongly from the tops of her thighbones down through her feet? Extending long through the spine and out through the top of the head? Radiating out from her heart center through her fingertips?

If you're facilitating this process with other teachers or trainees, this is an opportune time to address specific verbal cues and hands-on adjustments that reflect and thus address the observations. This process should include the clear sequencing of cues, how to combine verbal and physical cues, and where and how to demonstrate what you are cueing. Across the course of a workshop or training program, this can be done in round-robin style, with each participant taking turns giving what he or she sees as the most important cue, until the group has collectively guided the model student into and out of the asana.

Step 3: Practice Teaching Observation

Guided practice teaching is an integral component of any credible teacher-training program and an essential part of learning to see and guide students in their asana practice. Start by teaching a single asana to one other participant. Simulating the reality of an actual class, one partner takes the teacher role, and the other partner takes the student role. Using what you know (staying away from instructions you do not understand), guide your student into the asana. Go through the same process described above for asana laboratory observation, except that you are now observing *and* cueing. Start with purely verbal cues. As you become more comfortable in simultaneously observing and giving verbal cues, start to practice demonstrating while guiding your partner (we will cover demonstration below). Take your time (while honoring your partner's needs), staying attentive to what your partner is doing and giving verbal cues based on what you see and understand as the principles of the asana. Begin to weave verbal and physical cues together, always speaking to what you are encouraging with your physical cues.

As you progress from teaching one asana to one student to a few or several asanas to a small group, notice what happens to your observational practice, cues, and demonstrations. You will now experience seeing each student doing something slightly or very different from others in your group. Use this opportunity to hone

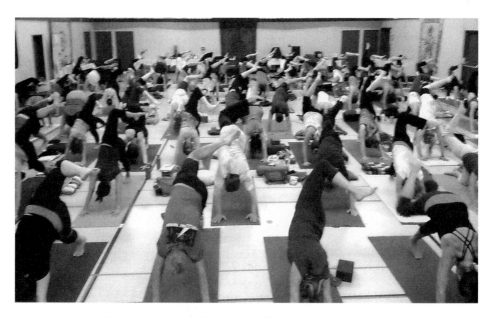

Observing students is more challenging in large classes.

your visual observation skills. Continue to give initial attention to the areas most at risk. Try to address those risks while maintaining your awareness of what is happening with others in your group. Notice the tendency to become so absorbed in something with one student that you momentarily lose sight and connection with everyone else. Here we come to a place where our personal practice of concentration and attention—being simultaneously focused and broadly aware—has tangible benefit in teaching.

Let your observational skills deepen as you progress into apprenticing and independent teaching. Apply them the moment you first meet and greet a new student. While doing the comprehensive observation described above, notice the student's natural posture as you ask about his or her background. One benefit of bringing a class into Tadasana (Mountain Pose) at or toward the beginning of class is that it allows you to easily observe students' basic posture. Then expand your observation asana by asana. Notice how the tendencies evident in Tadasana likely manifest in more pronounced form as students move into more complex asanas. Use this observation to further refine your subsequent understanding of how different asanas increase the challenges seen in the more basic positions.

Throughout this process of learning to see and relate to students, remember that you are teaching yoga, not trying to get people into poses. Keep coming back to the principle of yoga as a *practice of awareness and awakening,* not of attainment. Try to look at each student as the unique and beautiful person he or she is in the moment. Explore how you can share what you are seeing in a way that helps that student to see more easily and clearly and to feel his or her own body, breath, and practice. Remember the principles of sthira, sukham, asanam. Apply this to yourself while encouraging it in your students. Keep watching, keep breathing, feel your heart, and keep practicing your observational skills.

Further Approaching, Assessing, and Communicating with Students

As you move closer to giving hands-on guidance to your students, it's important to consider how to best approach, assess, and communicate with your students. Proceed with these three steps in further preparing to give hands-on assists and guidance:

1. **Look for inner and outer beauty first.** Many teachers rush to judgment in their observation of students, often leading them to see only what is

"wrong" rather than appreciating the intrinsic and extrinsic beauty of the student doing whatever they are doing in any asana. Find the beauty, and acknowledge it to yourself and to the student. This will help reinforce the idea that you are working with a real human being in an asana practice rather than a model posing for a camera, the former altogether real and the latter a contrived performance.

2. **Next, look at and address what, if anything, might be most at risk.** Ideally we address risk issues in giving the verbal cues and demonstrations that guide students into an asana and its modified or basic form. Still, many students will end up with positioning that could be injurious or otherwise problematic. As you observe the class transitioning in to an asana, watch primarily for how they are moving and positioning in relation to what is most at risk. If you see students who are not appearing to respond to your risk prevention–related cues, reinforce the cue verbally and with physical demonstration before offering a hands-on cue.

3. **Look for steadiness, ease, and presence of mind in the face, eyes, breath, and overall energetic presence.** The face, eyes, and breath provide instant sources of insight into how one is feeling and faring in an asana. Tension shows immediately in the face and eyes, and the eyes provide further insight into a student's focus in the practice. The breath also mirrors how one is doing energetically and further clarifies if a student is feeling stress or strain. Encourage modifications to make the asana sufficiently simple and accessible so that the student is calm, present, and thereby more capable of refining how they are doing what they are doing.

Qualities of Touch

How we touch is just as important as when and where. It is in how we touch that touching becomes a tool for teaching. The various qualities of touch offer different means of tactile communication in which both teacher and student are active participants in the student deepening his or her understanding and experience in the asana practice. Some qualities are decidedly subtler than others; the subtler the quality of touch, the more the student can be a consciously coactive participant in this shared experience. As discussed earlier, rather than adjusting students, in giving hands-on cues we are working with them one-on-one to guide and assist them in refining their practice in keeping with the intention and condition. Here are the basic ways we can best engage in this tactile form of communicating with students.

- **awakening or relaxing:** With awakening touch we can encourage muscular activation and cue-related directional intentions in the body. For example, lightly touching the top of the head in Tadasana while verbally cueing the student to press the head into your hand encourages a line of energy out through the top of the head, while pressing into the heel of the foot of the grounded leg in Supta Padangusthasana encourages extension and energetic engagement through that leg and heel. With each of the examples given above for clarifying touch, we can go further by apply-

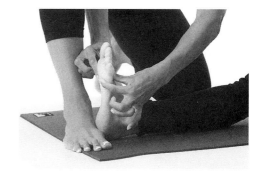
Awakening the foot and leg in Supta Padangusthasana (Reclined Big Toe Pose).

  ing more pressure to create awakening or relaxing cues, offering the pressure of our fingertips to the muscles in a way that allows the student to more fully feel the engagement or relaxation of the muscles.

- **clarifying:** This quality of touch allows you to ascertain whether or to what extent a student is activating certain muscles or engaging in certain energetic actions. For example, in Adho Mukha Svanasana, we want to encourage students to activate the quadriceps muscles as a means of stabilizing the legs and stimulating the reciproca-linnervation that tells the hamstrings to relax and lengthen; we can do this by lightly pressing into the quadriceps while asking the student to lift the knee cap, then observing to see and feel the reaction. With Urdhva Dhanurasana (Upward-Facing Bow Pose), we can apply clarifying touch in much the opposite way: to see if the upper fibers of the glutei maximi are relatively relaxed so that there is less pressure around the sacroiliac joint.

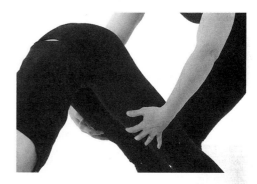
Clarifying the engagement of the quadriceps muscle in Adho Mukha Svanasana (Downward-Facing Dog Pose).

- **stabilizing:** While as a general principle of teaching we should always strive to help students toward independence, sometimes that goal is brought closer to reality through active support. Many asanas involve challenges to balance that become even more challenging when the teacher suggests a modification or variation. Here we can use our body to give the student added stability, giving only as much or as little as it takes to

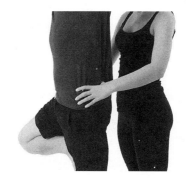
Stabilizing a student's balance in Vrksasana (Tree Pose).

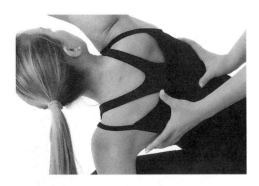

Emphasizing elongation and rotation in Utthita Parsvakonasana (Extended Side Angle Pose).

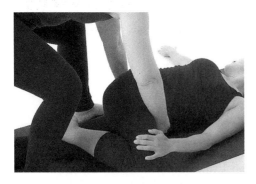

Moving a student to position his or her lower hip to center in Supta Parivartanasana (Reclined Revolved Pose).

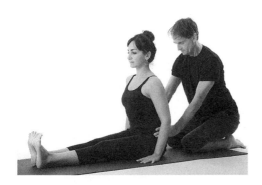

Grounding touch to keep a student's sitting bones rooted to the floor in Paschimottanasana (West Stretching Pose or Seated Forward Fold).

accomplish that purpose. For example, you could place your hip lightly yet stably against a student's hip in Ardha Chandrasana (Half Moon Pose) or Vrksasana to help keep the student balanced while using your hands to offer other physical cues.

- **emphasizing:** Slightly more suggestive or directive than awakening or relaxing touch, in giving emphasizing touch we offer a light surface cue to encourage a specific movement, such as elongation and rotation of the torso in Utthita Parsvakonasana. Here we can apply more or less tactile pressure depending on what we feel or otherwise perceive in the student's reaction. The intention with this quality of touch is both to help the student better understand the dynamics of stability, ease, and movement in the asana (or in transition in or out of it) and to suggest how he or she might better refine positioning or energetic action.

- **moving:** If we give clear verbal cues and demonstrations, then we should only fairly rarely find ourselves needing to help a student with a fundamental repositioning of their body. Generally, the better approach is to ask the student to come out of the asana in order to approach it anew with attention to the desired positioning. When we do reposition part of the body in a significant way, we are achieving a change in basic alignment. For example, in Jathara Parivartanasana (Revolving Twist Pose), many students will not shift the lower hip to the midline of their mat while transitioning into this asana, consequently creating something of a back bend through the spine that detracts from the truer twist this asana otherwise creates. The moving touch in this example involves picking up the student and bringing his or her lower hip to center.

- **grounding:** The effort to go farther or deeper in an asana often compromises its foundation, which consequently introduces likelier strain. With grounding touch, we press part of the body down to enhance the foundation of an asana, thereby enabling the student to explore more safely. For example, many students will so strongly attempt to pull their torso forward in Paschimottanasana that the sitting bones lose their active rooting, compromising space in the lumbar spine while creating more pressure against intervertebral disks and tension in the lumbar ligaments. Pressing firmly down on the back of the pelvis (on the ilia) will give the student rooting that allows greater elongation of the spine.

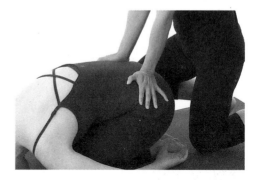

Comforting a student in Balasana (Child's Pose).

- **comforting:** Giving comforting human contact can convey emotional support and compassion. For example, simply resting your hand on a student's back in Balasana can suggest deeper relaxation and offer a sense of caring. In giving comforting touch it is important to have clear intention and action so that the touch is comforting rather than inappropriately sensual.

How Not to Touch

Knowing how to touch is important; knowing how not to touch is of utmost importance. While knowing how to touch provides clues and insights about how not to touch, there is a tendency among many yoga teachers to be less than clear or committed to appreciating the importance of staying in the realm of informed and appropriate physical cueing. Here we look at several types of common hands-on contact that are not appropriate.

- **distally:** In chapter 2 we discussed the importance of working with safe biomechanics, including by giving students proximal adjustments. Giving a distal adjustment in which you cue or create movement by clasping and moving a student's arm or leg from their hand or foot is simply unnecessary and fraught with danger to hypermobile or impinged joints. The distal clasp creates excessive leverage. Thus, clasping the upper hand in Utthita Trikonasana (Extended Triangle Pose) to reposition the arm can cause subluxation of the shoulder. Pressing down on the hands in Prasarita Padottanasana C (Spread-Leg Forward Fold Pose C) creates excessive leverage against the shoulder joint while causing greater hyperextension in the elbow of students with hypermobility challenges. Pulling back on the shoulders in Urdhva Mukha Svanasana (Upward-Facing Dog Pose) or Bhujangasana (Cobra Pose) is distal to the lumbar spine and can cause injury to the lower back.

- **forcefully:** In playing the edge within and between asanas, students are ideally attuned to the breath as a primary source of self-guided practice that honors their own intention while cultivating steadiness and ease. All of this can be undermined with a forceful adjustment, or worse yet, the force can cause an injury as a student is pushed, pulled, or rotated beyond their safe range of motion. A common forceful adjustment is found when a teacher helps a student to wrap and clasp something in asanas such as Marichyasana C (Sage Marichi's Pose C) or the wrapped variations of Ardha Matsyendrasana (Half Lord of the Fishes Pose) or Utthita Parsvakonasana. The forceful assistance in each of these examples can easily strain the labrum around the shoulder and the ligaments along the lumbar spine.

- **meanderingly:** Our hands-on cues should be specific and deliberate. When we wander around with our hands due to our own confusion or from being lackadaisical, the student we are touching is likely to become confused and consequently taken out of their focused practice. The most common cause of a meandering cue is uncertainty about what one is intending with the cue and how best to accomplish that intention. Teaching what you know and not guessing in the middle of teaching to the best of your knowledge, you will simply not give an adjustment until you know your intention and how to fulfill it (all evolving in the moment as you connect with the student in the communicative process of it all).

- **blindly:** Part of the art of teaching is staying fully present to what you are doing. In giving tactile guidance, it is important to pay attention to the student you are working with, even if you are multitasking in staying aware of what is happening with other students in the class. As you begin to place your hands on a student and then give whatever cue you are offering, at that moment, stay fully present to the student and your adjustment to see and feel what you are doing and how your student is responding. If you attempt to give blind guidance, your cues will very likely be unhelpful and probably confusing; worse yet, giving blind adjustments, you are more likely to press on vulnerable joints or organs and to inadvertently touch inappropriately.

- **destabilizing:** Sometimes our best intentions as a teacher can create problems for our students. While intentionally offering students stabilizing support, we can easily cause just the opposite. For example, in giving added support to a student's balance in Parivrtta Trikonasana while cueing elongation and rotation of the spine, teachers commonly and unconsciously cause the student to become dependent on them for their overall balance; as the teacher steps away from the student, the student tends to lose stable balance and may even fall. This is primarily about focused awareness: in balance-sensitive asanas, bring more awareness to giving very light support to the balance aspect (as much or as little contact and pressure as it takes) while giving whatever other cues you might, and even more awareness to any shift in the student's balance as you gradually relax your contact with him or her.

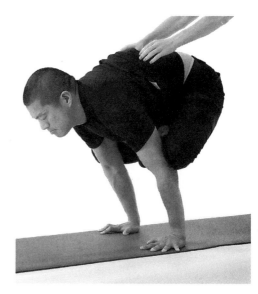

It is easy to destabilize a student in balance-sensitive asanas like Urdhva Kukkutasana (Upward Rooster Pose).

- **randomly:** Similar to meandering touch but perhaps more intentional, random touch involves giving cues with no particular logic or order, instead based more on whim (which sometimes arrogantly masquerades as intuition). Also like meandering cues, they are confusing and distracting. Understanding the fundamentals of the asana, attuned to the student you are with, you will give cues that make sense to the student as he or she explores the asana from its foundation up.

- **inappropriately:** The term *inappropriate* is broadly inclusive of touch that is not based on clear understanding of alignment, safe biomechanics, or crossing personal boundaries with overly sensuous or sexual touch. Consider not just where you touch, but how. You will know if the quality of touch is inappropriate by measuring it against your purpose as a teacher in supporting students in their practices.

Self-Preservation and Teacher Positioning

It is common for teachers to lose their own grounding and comfort when working with their students. By staying grounded and attentive to your own stability and ease, you are better able to guide and support your students. Positioning yourself in a way that is stable and comfortable, then moving into the adjustment with a feeling of your own stability and ease, will help ensure that you do not hurt yourself while helping students. This requires being especially attuned to your lower back, wrists, and parts of your body that are either strained or more susceptible to injury. Keep your knees bent when giving standing assists. The relative size of your body and those of your students will be a significant factor in your positioning. You may find yourself standing, kneeling, sitting down, or positioning yourself in other ways that allow you to work most stably and easily while staying attuned to your student. Rather than adopting a specific stance for each and every adjustment, be open to playing around with how you position your own body to take care of yourself while giving active assistance to your students. Try to give tactile assistance with your wrists in neutral extension and some simple wrist stretches throughout each class to keep your wrists healthy and happy.

Five Basic Steps in Giving Hands-On Cues and Assistance

As we discussed earlier, hands-on cues and assistance are one of several methods of giving instructional guidance to students. To the extent that you give clear verbal cues combined with effective demonstrations, most students will not need tactile cues. To make your cues most effective, speak slowly while simultaneously moving slowly into the asana you are teaching, giving slightly dramatic emphasis to whatever you most want to highlight while transitioning in from a position in which you mirror your class with maximum visual contact between you and all of your students. Try not to say what *not* to do; instead, emphasize what *to* do. (Saying what not to do often confuses students, especially if they miss the "not" part of your instruction.) Try to order your verbal cues as discussed in detail in chapter 4 of *Yoga Sequencing*. Try to verbally cue to what you are seeing students doing or not doing as they transition into the asana, and give them a chance to physically express the cue before rushing to their aid.

When demonstrating, mirror your students in a way that maximizes their view of you and your view of them. In doing so, further observe your students to determine what further or clearer guidance is most needed. Appreciate that even the most adept yoga student may sense that they have positioned their body in accordance with what you've instructed and demonstrated, yet in reality they might be far from it. Other less experienced or adept students as well as more purely tactile learners may reveal that they can benefit from tactile guidance from the beginning of your instruction. Otherwise, once you've completed your demonstration, it's time to get off your mat and out into the room to better observe your students and perhaps offer the more refined guidance that appears to be needed. When teaching, teach. Do your personal practice another time.

To best engage with the student in a mutually interactive way, provide light contact on the places where you are verbally cueing the movement and give a verbal cue for the student to breath and move into the light pressure that you are giving in equal proportion to the student's movement into your point of contact. As a general method to assist the student in playing the edge in the asanas, always cue backing slightly away from where he or she can comfortably go on each inhalation, then on the exhalations cue and encourage the student to move slightly farther in whatever ways are being cued. By maintaining contact while asking the student to breathe into the light resistance you are giving with your tactile cue, he or she can most easily feel and create the suggested movements in gradually refining the asana. This method is given more nuanced explanation and examples in each of the five basic steps in giving tactile support.

Step 1: Stabilizing and Easing

The first priority in hands-on teaching is to help ensure that students are steady and at ease in their practice. As with all other aspects of asana instruction, this starts with verbal cues and demonstration. Once you determine that hands-on assistance will be helpful, and the student agrees, your initial focus should address any risk issues that could lead to injury or complicate a preexisting condition. As most problems of unease arise from a faulty foundation, once you have addressed basic risk issues, give your attention to properly (or further) establishing the foundation of the asana. This may involve complete repositioning (asking the student to come out of the asana and begin anew), use of props, and modifications that set up the foundation of the asana for that particular student in a different way than you cued for the larger class. With the foundation established, give hands-on cues— using the grounding quality of touch—to accentuate the student's rooting action. Whenever the grounding action is not primarily down into the floor, provide a point of resistance against which the student can press.

For example, if the student is lying supine in Supta Padangusthasana, place your foot or hand against the student's heel while verbally cueing her to press against your point of contact, meeting and going with the student's intentional effort to encourage the comfortable and sustainable maximum mutual pressure. Then, working in synchrony with the student's breathing patterns, physically and verbally cue the relationship between roots, breath, and ease by maintaining your grounding action cue and highlighting the spaciousness that happens with the inhalations, and the deeper release and ease that happens with the exhalations.

Bring renewed attention to the breath by highlighting the same qualities of steadiness and ease in the flow of the breath itself, encouraging a manifold connection between the qualities of breath and bodymind.

Step 2: Elongating the Spine

Keeping the spine in mind, next focus on working from the foundation of the asana to cultivate more space, especially up along the entire length of the spine. Here you are cueing the connection between roots and extension. While remaining attentive to the foundation of the asana, again work with the flow of the student's breath to physically and verbally cue elongation of the spine: with the student's inhalation, encourage expansion and elongation from the roots of the asana up along the spine; with the exhalation, encourage maintenance of that spaciousness along with a feeling of release and ease. Offer a point of light contact on top of the student's head while cueing the student to elongate up into it. In asanas such as Sirsasana (Headstand), make this contact on the feet to similarly cue elongation of the spine and the entire body. With most students, this will involve an accentuating quality of touch in which your hands are suggesting the continuous elongation of the spine without compromising steadiness or ease. Amid this guidance you have the perfect situation to give added emphasis to heart-centered breathing, further enhancing spaciousness and a connection to one's intention in the practice.

Step 3: Rotating, Flexing, and Extending the Spine

Elongating the spine is the essential preparation for rotating, flexing, or extending it. Many students will attempt to twist, fold forward, or bend back before maximizing the comfortable lengthening of their spine, which makes any of those former movements less internally inviting, more difficult, and more likely to both limit range of motion and increase the likelihood of strain. Working from the foundation of the asana, always cue elongation of the spine with the inhalations (which helps to create space), maintenance of that space with the exhalations, and gradual movement into initial rotation, flexion, or extension of the spine also with exhalations. The cueing applies a few different qualities of touch: grounding, emphasizing, and light moving. This is a continuous, dynamic process that should be cued in synchrony with the student's breathing pattern: inhaling, root and elongate (while backing slightly away from any rotation, flexion, or extension); exhaling, rotate, fold, or extend farther. In all of these cues, use the method of mutual pressure while cueing the student to breathe into the point of contact you are providing, maintaining dynamic contact in which the student is better feeling what it takes to move in the cued ways.

Step 4: Refining the Asana

The first three steps establish the basic elements of the asana. Exploring from this foundation, next begin to cue its further refinement to help instill a sense of equanimity amid the intensity of the experience. Rather than thinking that this takes the asana into a deeper or more complex form, let refinement be about making it simpler in the basics of roots, extension, and whatever other energetic actions are involved in the particular asana. Verbally guide the student to refocus on the breath to renew its steady, balanced flow, to soften the eyes amid the steadiness of the gaze, and to tune in to find more subtle ways of making the asana feel natural while continuing to be with it in a way that feels significant. Remember: persevering practice *abhyasa* and nonattachment *vairagya*. Now let your hands-on guidance go to the aspects of the asana that might be sources of this refining exploration, your tactile guidance now using more clarifying and emphasizing qualities of touch. Keep your student coming back to connecting breath and movement, breath and sensation, breath and awareness in the bodymind.

Step 5: Deepening the Asana

With the essential elements of the asana manifesting and more refined expression of it coming through the steadiness and ease of the breath, encourage deeper exploration without losing the essential qualities already established. Deepening the asana may involve simply staying with it longer while continuing to explore its refinement. It may also involve going further with it, including with variations that introduce new elements. Note that attempting variations that take an asana deeper makes no sense prior to the first four steps given here. Rather, rushing ahead to vary or otherwise deepen the expression of the asana is likely to undermine its integrity, disrupt the yogic process of consciously connecting breath-bodymind, and create a more likely path to injury than to something beneficial. Reserve your deepening hands-on assistance for students who appear to have taken the wise progression of steps 1 through 4, and encourage anyone who is straining to back off, slow down, and stay in the practice. Remind your students that it is not about how *far* one goes, but *how* one goes.

Yoga Adjustment Positioning and Techniques

The qualities of touch discussed earlier give us general sensitivities we can tap into when working with our students. Here we look at specific hands-on techniques and offer examples to elucidate each one. These techniques will vary based on you—particularly your intentions, your height relative to a student, the size of your hands, and the relative dimensions and conditions of the student you are cueing. There are innumerable variations and permutations of these positioning options and touching techniques that are presented in part II, including many that make creative use of other parts of the body. All can be played with to find what works best for you in guiding the unique students in your classes.

Physical Stances

How you position yourself is important for your own well-being and for giving the best possible assistance. There are three basic stances than can and should be varied depending on the specific assist and the needs and dimensions of you and your students: standing, kneeling, and sitting. Here are three examples of each stance:

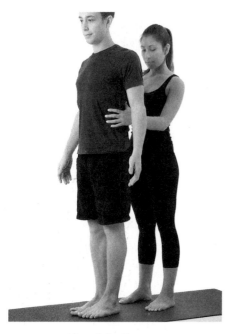

Mountain Stance.

Mountain Stance involves standing with both legs straight, as one does in Tadasana. Depending on your height and the height of the student you are assisting, the legs are kept fully extended, feet hip distance apart, with variations in foot position to enhance stability.

In **Horse Stance** the feet are separated two to three feet apart and the knees are bent, providing a stable foundation, ease in the lower back, and more powerful leveraging when pushing with the arms and hands.

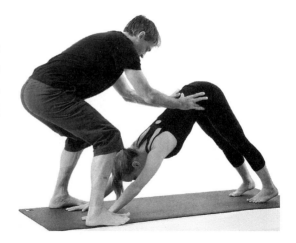

Horse Stance.

Hip Stance allows the use of one hip against the hip, back, or shoulder of a student to help stabilize the student's balance and basic positioning while encouraging refinement elsewhere in the asana (such as elongation of the spine or rotation of the torso or arm).

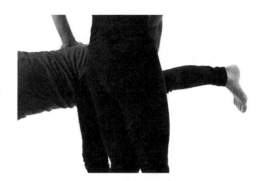

Hip Stance.

One Knee Down Stance is a kneeling position that allows you to work more effectively at your mid-height. This positioning is effective for working at mid-height with students in standing asanas, depending on your height relative to theirs'. This stance has many applications, including in standing asanas such as Virabhadrasana II (Warrior II Pose), where you can use the hip of your non-kneeling side to help stabilize the student's hip position.

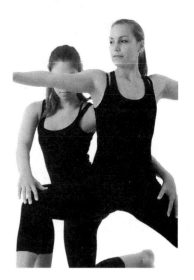

One Knee Down Stance.

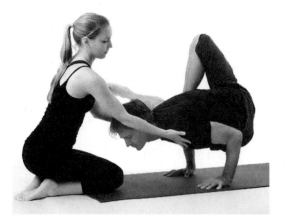

Knees Down Stance.

With the knees on the floor and the feet either extended back or toes curled under, the **Knees Down Stance** gives you stability and good leverage when working with students in many seated asanas and other asanas in which the focus of your assistance is approximately two feet above the floor.

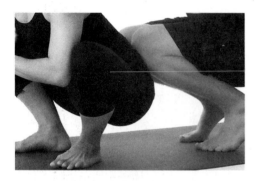

Low Chair Stance.

Low Chair Stance is akin to the original form of Utkatasana (Chair Pose) as described in the Hatha Yoga Pradipika. In this variation of that asana, the toes are curled under, the heels lifted, and the knees and hands are used for giving the assistance. Generally this positioning is used to slide the knees up the quadratus lumborum muscles in asanas such as Baddha Konasana (Bound Angle Pose) or Malasana (Garland Pose). Depending on the positioning and flexibility of the student, the knees can slide farther up the lower back *(not on the spine),* thus bringing the shins into play at the point of pressure to the sides of the student's spine (initially still on the quadratus lumborum muscles, and possibly sliding farther up to the sides of the spine).

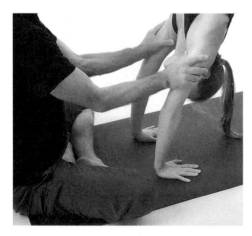

Simply Sitting Stance.

Simply Sitting Stance brings the teacher to the floor and makes it easier to give assistance to students in many seated and supine positions. It is best used when giving light cues and there is little need for leveraged pressure.

Akin to Virasana (Hero Pose), except sitting off to the sides of the heels as one would in setting up for Bharadvajrasana A (Sage Bharadvaj's Pose A), **Noose Stance** is useful for positioning in closer to the student in asymmetrical asanas in which the physical assists are best given from behind.

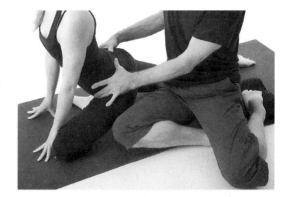

Noose Stance.

Wide Leg Stance is essentially an upright Upavista Konasana (Wide-Angle Forward Fold Pose) in which there is the option of using the weight of the legs to accentuate the student's grounding of the legs while using the hands to cue other actions.

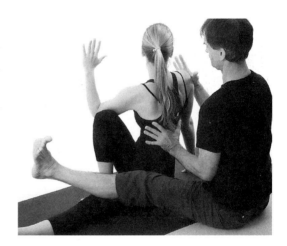

Wide Leg Stance.

Hand Positions and Movements

With **Hip Handles,** the hands are placed around the back of the pelvis with the thumbs pointing toward the sacrum and the fingers wrapped outward around the posterior superior iliac spines. This enables you to simultaneously cue the grounding of the sitting bones and the anterior rotation of the pelvis in nearly all seated asanas.

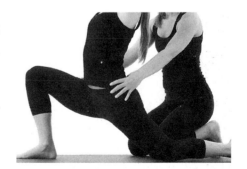

Hip Handles.

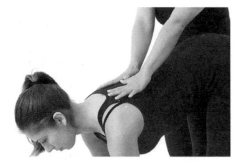

Open Palms.

With the **Open Palms** position, we spread and fully extend the fingers to create a wide-open palm that is most often applied in movement-oriented assists. The open palm provides a direct source of contact, while the extended fingers give more focused energy to the palmar contact with the student. It is the ideal hand positioning when assisting most twists and has multiple other applications.

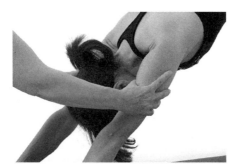 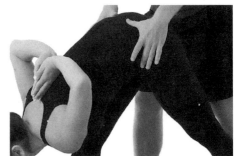

Clasping Rotation.

Clasping Rotation is an emphasizing, stabilizing, or moving cue applied proximally to the arms or thighs to accentuate rotation of the appendage. If done strongly, it is important to cue stability in the torso-shoulder girdle when working with the arms or the pelvis when working with the legs.

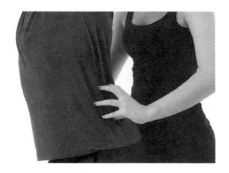

Finger Spread.

The **Finger Spread** starts with the fingertips drawn relatively toward each other before extending and abducting the fingers in encouraging more space, such as in the uniform lengthening of the lower rim of the rib cage up and away from the upper rim of the pelvis, thus creating more space through the lumbar spine. See the section on Tadasana in chapter 4 for an example of this cue when assisting students.

In contrast to the Finger Spread, with the **Finger Draw** we are cueing with the opposite movement of the fingertips, starting with the fingers spread wide apart and then drawing them toward the opposing thumb tips to encourage more space in the areas from which the fingertips are moving away. This cue is usefully applied with the fingertips across the superior border of the scapula and the thumb tips positioned as far down the scapulae as possible to create more space around the neck in asanas in which the shoulder blades tend to elevate and create compression around the neck.

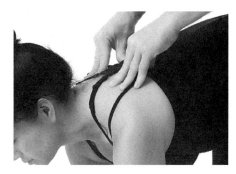

Finger Draw.

Opposite Rotation enables you to simultaneously cue opposing actions across a joint. With appendicular cues, it is generally given in conjunction with a stabilizing or moving cue on or closer to the axial skeleton, accentuating rotation without losing the alignment or energetic actions of the more proximal or axial part of the body in asanas such as Upavista Konasana or Baddha Konasana. It is equally useful in encouraging fuller extension of the thoracic spine,

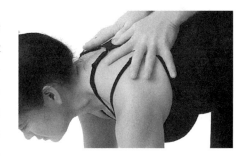

Opposite Rotation.

and with it a more spacious heart center, by simultaneously cueing the sternum forward and shoulder blades down against the back ribs in most forward folding asanas (see the section on Ardha Uttanasana in chapter 4 for an example of this cue when assisting students).

Light **Finger Flicks** effectively cue certain energetic actions with an accentuating or awakening quality of touch. It is similar to the Finger Spread, except it is done with a flicking action to better suggest activation. Here we see an example of this cue applied to the medial arches of the feet, where the intention is to awaken pada bandha.

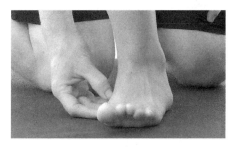

Finger Flicks.

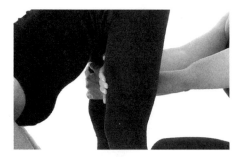

Crossed Wrists.

Crossed Wrists position enables you to cue internal rotation of the thighs with an emphasizing quality of touch. It is most commonly applied from behind in Adho Mukha Svanasana, where by crossing the wrists, clasping around the thighs, and then pulling back, you both internally rotate the femurs and accentuate the elongation of the spine.

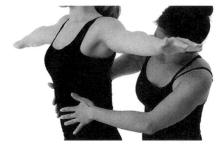

Light Hands.

Light Hands refers to a variety of specific hand positions in which you intuitively apply the hands with very light pressure, such as cueing the floating ribs to draw slightly in when in Tadasana.

Departing a Student

It is important to give just as much awareness to how you depart a student as you give to how you first approach a student. With all instances of hands-on assistance, begin your departure by giving your student a sense that you are letting go. In letting go, do so gradually in order to help ensure student stability, your own stability and ease, and to facilitate the student coming gracefully back to being in whatever he or she is doing with greater autonomy. This is especially important in asanas involving balance or intense physical and energetic engagement, where a sudden change in pressure can cause unintended movement.

How you depart should be further informed by several factors, including the qualities of the specific asana, whether the student will remain in the asana or transition out with your assistance, the time given in the assistance, your sense of the student's condition as you begin to release contact, and your own well-being. To begin, consider how dependent the student is on your support. The more dependent, the more gradually you should release contact while communicating verbally to help ensure a common sense of what is happening and about to happen. This is an important consideration in any assistance in which the student is now relatively dependent on you for support. The following two contrasting examples highlight the dependence-release dynamic:

- Balance can be challenging in Parivrtta Trikonasana, and in giving assistance, it is almost impossible not to affect it. Thus, as you begin to let go, it is important to get a sense of the student's stability, giving light tapping contact to gently cue the student toward centered balance as they come back under their own exclusive control.

- When moving a student beyond the range of motion that they are capable of creating for themselves, especially in contraction back bends such as Salabhasana A (Locust Pose A), letting go of the support you are giving will cause them to drop down to the point where they do have muscular control, which in this example can cause a stretch reflex in the spinal erector muscles in which sudden gripping of those muscles can cause strain. When supporting a student beyond his or her self-controlled range of motion, always ease them back to being within their own control, and only then gradually release your support.

If your assistance will continue through the transition out of an asana, consider giving support to the transitional movement in a way that helps highlight the energetic actions that will make the movement safer and easier. Here are three examples to highlight the value of this transitional support with three very different asanas:

- **Utthita Trikonasana:** Muscles supporting the lower back are asked to work strongly when transitioning back to standing upright. Instructing students to run a stronger line of energy from the back hip to the back foot will make this transition easier on the lower back. Cue this action by placing a hand on the lateral side of the superior pelvis and give a grounding quality of touch that emphasizes rooting from that hip to the heel as the student is coming up.

- **Paschimottanasana** and most other seated forward folds: The issue here is similar to the example given with Utthita Trikonasana: raising the torso from a folded or laterally extended position without straining the lower back. Here the hand placement is the same as given in providing a grounding quality of assistance to the pelvis in this asana, as shown in the section on Paschimottanasana in chapter 9. As the student inhales to slowly rise, use the grounding cue at the pelvis along with a rotational cue to encourage steady rooting of the sitting bones and posterior rotation of the pelvis as the primary source of drawing the torso to vertical.

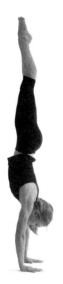

- **Adho Mukha Vrksasana** (Downward-Facing Tree Pose or Handstand): If you assisted a student in getting into a handstand, assist him or her in coming back down. The assistance should be twofold: easing the transition of the feet back to the floor, and then suggesting staying in a standing forward fold for at least a few breaths prior to standing up in order to prevent orthostatic hypotension (dizziness and possible fainting).

While many cues are given for just a few seconds (especially clarifying or awakening cues), others may involve prolonged support. The longer you assist a student, the more gradually you should release contact. Depending on the overall needs of the class, longer holds may also require further explanation or conversation with the student in order to make clearer the purpose of the assistance, to draw out the student's experience of it, and to gain insight into how the student (and you as the teacher) might refine the practice when next approaching that or a similar asana.

Lastly, it is important to consider the student's and your own overall condition in how you depart a student. Try to be as informed as you can about any condition that might affect the ease with which a student comes out of an asana. If you are giving assistance to the transition, include your own condition in that consideration, and take care of yourself so you are better able to give appropriate and mutually comfortable support to the student and to yourself.

Part II
Applications

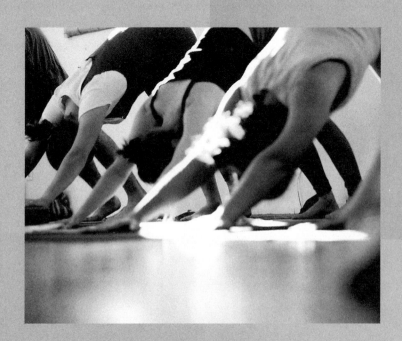

Chapter 4

Standing Asanas

STANDING ASANAS ARE THE POWERFULLY GROUNDING PHYSICAL FOUNDATION for the overall asana practice. Standing on their feet, students begin to experience how a stable foundation creates support up through their legs, pelvis, spine, arms, and head. They also discover that a stable foundation is resilient, beginning with the activation of pada bandha in the feet. Blending sthira and sukham in the standing asanas, students begin to find samasthihi (equal standing), which invokes an attitude and awareness of equanimity as they feel the connection of body, breath, mind, and spirit. In deepening this sense of equanimity, students develop an embodied awareness of how the lightness of being depends on being grounded, allowing them to move about in their yoga practice and daily life with greater ease and joy.

Standing asanas are divided into three categories: (1) externally rotated femurs, (2) neutrally or internally rotated femurs, and (3) standing balance asanas. Externally rotated standing asanas generally stretch the inner groin and thighs while strengthening the external rotators and abductors. Internally rotated standing asanas generally strengthen the adductors and internal rotators while stretching the external rotators and abductors. (Neutral rotation is close to internal rotation in its actions and effects, but the rotational effort is very slight.) Standing balance asanas strengthen the entire standing leg and the pelvic girdle while creating an opportunity to explore the instinctual fear of falling while moving into steadier balance.

Taken together, these asanas teach us about the integration of practice as we discover how the feet are connected to the legs, pelvis, spine, heart center, head, and arms—and ultimately to the breath and sense of embodied awakening. Following initial warming and awakening movements such as Cat and Dog Tilts, Surya Namaskara (Sun Salutation), or kapalabhati pranayama, standing asanas are the safest asana family for warming and opening the entire body in preparation for more complex asanas. Standing asanas are energetically stimulating, helping to focus the mind and awaken the body in the early part of the practice.

An Awakened Foundation

Activation of the feet begins in the legs as we run lines of energy from the top of our femur bones down through our feet. This creates a "rebouncing effect." Imagine the feeling of being heavier when riding up in an elevator, or lighter when riding down. The pressure of the elevator floor up against your feet not only makes you feel heavier, it has the effect of causing the muscles in your legs to engage more strongly. Similarly, when you intentionally root down from the tops of your thighbones down into your feet, the muscles in your calves and thighs engage. This not only creates the upward pull on the arches of pada bandha (primarily from the stirrup-like effect of activating the tibialis posterior and peroneus longus muscles) but creates expansion through the joints and a sense of being more firmly grounded yet resilient in your feet while longer, lighter, and more integrated up through your body. To more fully cultivate pada bandha, guide your students as follows:

- Bring the class to standing with their feet together at the front of their mat.
- Ask them to look down at their feet and lift and spread their toes wide apart.
- Keeping the toes lifted, guide your students to feel the inner edges of the balls of their feet (about an inch in from the space between the big toe and the second toe) and to press that point more firmly down into the floor.
- Now ask students to repeatedly release the toes down and lift them up while keeping the inner edges of the balls of their feet rooting down,

noticing how this stimulates the awakening and lifting of the inner arches and ankles.

- Encourage the class to try to keep their inner arches and ankles lifted and to feel how this creates a sense of lifting the center of each foot like a pyramid, creating pada bandha. The challenge arises in trying to maintain this awakening of the feet while allowing the toes to release softly down and spread into the floor, which becomes more natural and easier the more one practices it.
- Encourage students to maintain pada bandha in all standing asanas.

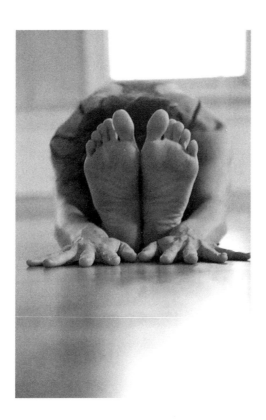

Tadasana (Mountain Pose)

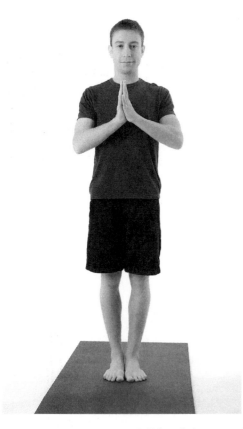

Tadasana is the foundational asana for all other standing asanas. As with all standing asanas, teach Tadasana from the ground up:

Give instructions for pada bandha and teach the importance of balancing the weight equally among the front, back, inside, and outside of each foot. With pada bandha active, instruct the contraction of the quadriceps along with the slight internal rotation of the femurs while pressing the femurs back, emphasizing how the internal rotation eases discovery of pelvic neutrality while broadening the space between the sitting bones.

Note that most students tend to tilt the pelvis anteriorly, which compresses the lower back and can lead to disk problems. A practice of opening and strengthening of the hip flexors, hip extensors, and abdominal core will help students move into stable pelvic neutrality. Guide students into feeling the connection between pada bandha and *mula bandha,* encouraging them to maintain mula bandha throughout their asana practice, lightly and without bearing down.

With pelvic neutrality, the spine will come into its natural curvature (neutral extension) in most students, unless there is significant muscular imbalance or a pathological condition such as scoliosis or kyphosis. Guide students into the light abdominal engagement that occurs naturally with complete exhalations, emphasizing how this helps to stabilize and lengthen the lumbar spine. The belly should be supple and stable. Cue the further lengthening of the spine by encouraging lifting the lower rim of the ribs up and away from the upper rim of the pelvis while allowing the floating ribs to soften naturally into the body.

Cue students to lift and broaden the sternum from inside while allowing the shoulder blades to draw lightly down and against the back ribs, further accentuating an expansive heart center while stabilizing the shoulders and creating ease in the neck. Instruct the broadening of the collarbones by first lifting the shoulders toward the ears, then drawing them back and down without losing the alignment in the lower- and mid-thoracic areas of the spine.

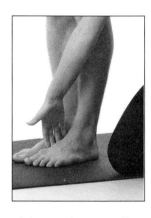

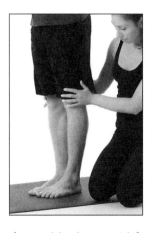

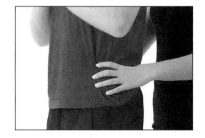

Use Light Hands to cue alignment of the feet and Finger Flicks to cue pada bandha as part of active grounding and equal standing (samasthihi).

For leg positioning, use Light Hands to cue the knees to point straight forward toward the centers of the feet.

Use Hip Handles with Clasping Rotation to cue pelvic neutrality in relation to the spine.

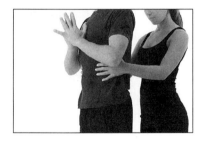

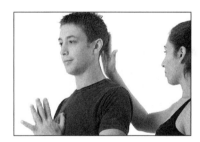

Use Light Hands to cue neutral positioning of the spine in its natural curvature, noting the tendency for students to either collapse or overly expand across the chest

Refine the positioning of the neck and head by instructing students to feel the positioning of their ears in line with their shoulders, then to draw the chin very slightly forward and down, lengthening the back of the neck while lifting through the throat. Finally, cue opening the crown of the head to the sky.

Explore Further

Teaching Yoga: pages 159-60

Yoga Sequencing: page 430

Teaching Yoga Resource Center:
   www.markstephensyoga.com/resources

Utkatasana (Chair Pose)

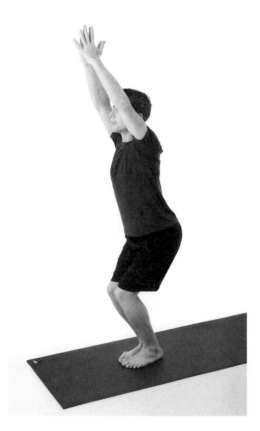

In instructing Utkatasana, ask students to place their hands into the creases of the groin, push the femoral heads toward the heels, and then rotate the pelvis forward and back a few times to find where it feels like the spine is drawing naturally out of their pelvis. Maintaining this pelvic neutrality, instruct them to release their arms down by their sides, turn their palms strongly out, and feel their chest expanding as their shoulder blades draw down and in and against their back ribs. Cue the class to reach their arms out and up overhead with an inhalation, keeping their shoulder blades rooting down as they stretch up through their chest and arms. Students can keep their arms shoulder distance apart and their gaze slightly down, or, with ease in the neck, toward the horizon. If they can keep their arms straight, invite them to draw their palms together and gaze up to their thumbs. Play around with guiding your classes from Tadasana to Utkatasana and back to Tadasana several times, emphasizing the connection of breath to movement, pada bandha to mula bandha, roots to extension up through the spine and arms. In the regular flow of Surya Namaskara B, transition from Utkatasana to Uttanasana (Standing Forward Bend Pose) by exhaling the legs straight while swan-diving forward and down. From Uttanasana, follow the same sequence from Surya Namaskara A to Adho Mukha Svanasana (Downward-Facing Dog Pose).

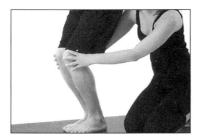

If the feet are placed together, use Light Touch to cue the knees to press together. If the feet are apart, use Light Touch to cue the feet forward over the centers of the feet.

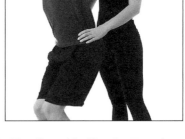

Use Hip Handles with Clasping Rotation to cue the student's pelvis forward and back until it is in neutral alignment with the lumbar spine.

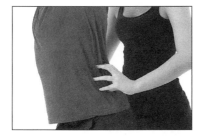

Use Finger Spreads to cue lifting the ribs away from the hips, thereby reducing pressure in the lower back.

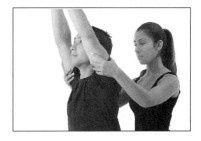

Use Clasping Rotation of the upper arms to encourage external rotation, flexion, and adduction of the arms at the shoulders.

Modification

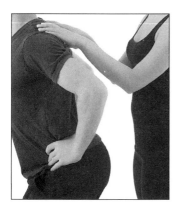

In first practicing Chair Pose, keep the hands on the hips to focus on pelvic neutrality while lifting up through the spine and rooting the shoulder blades down against the back ribs and expanding the chest.

Variation

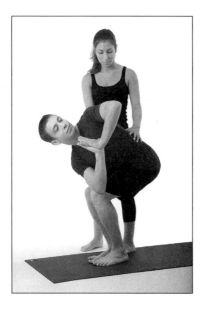

Introduce Parivrtta Utkatasana (Revolved Chair Pose) by verbally cueing and demonstrating drawing the right hand to the right hip, stretching the left arm toward the sky to lengthen along that side, then drawing the left elbow to the right knee and the palms together to encourage the twist, keeping the knees even with each other so the hips are level and there is less pressure in the lower back. If pressing the palms together strains the wrists, make one or both hands like fists or press the fingertips together. Over time, the shoulder may cross the knee, allowing that hand to release to the floor and the other arm to reach up, or wrap and clasp around the backs of the legs.

Explore Further

Teaching Yoga: page 171

Yoga Sequencing: page 442

Teaching Yoga Resource Center:
   www.markstephensyoga.com/resources

Ardha Uttanasana (Half Standing Forward Bend Pose)

Emphasize lengthening the spine, drawing the shoulder blades down the back, and further expanding across the heart center while drawing the sternum forward toward the horizon. Offer and demonstrate the options of having the knees bent, coming up onto the fingertips, and/or placing the hands high up on the shins. All of these options help to fully extend the spine. As students further develop the flexibility in the hamstrings and hips, cue them to keep their feet grounded and legs firm, thereby cultivating a more stable foundation from which to lengthen the spine.

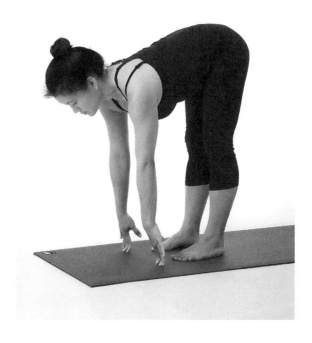

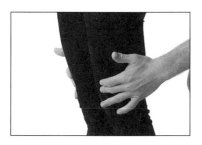

Starting in Tadasana or full Uttanasana, use a Light Hand above the knees to clarify or awaken engagement of the quadriceps muscles.

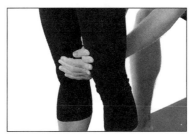

Use Crossed Wrists at mid-thigh to cue internal rotation of the thighs.

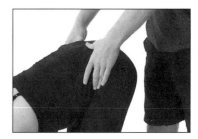

Use Clasping Rotation to cue anterior rotation of the pelvis as the initial and primary source of the forward fold while verbally cueing sensitivity to the lower back and hamstrings.

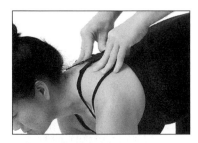

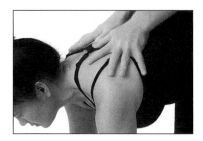

If the shoulders are shrugged toward the neck, use a light Finger Draw to cue the shoulder blades down against the back ribs.

With Open Palms placed wide across the shoulder blades, adduct the hands, giving an Opposite Rotation cue: thumbs cue the medial scapulae down the back while fingers cue extension of the chest forward.

Modification

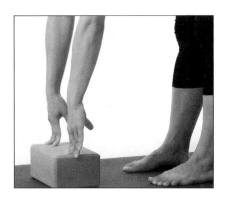

Prepare for full Ardha Uttanasana by placing the hands on a chair or blocks, at first keeping the knees slightly bent to take it easier on the lower back and the backs of the legs.

Explore Further

Teaching Yoga: page 161

Yoga Sequencing: page 368

Teaching Yoga Resource Center:
  www.markstephensyoga.com/resources

Uttanasana (Standing Forward Bend Pose)

Always offer the option of bending the knees to reduce stress on the hamstrings and the lower back. As students find comfort in the hamstrings and lower back, encourage them to focus more on activating their feet, keeping their legs firm, knee caps lifted, spine long, shoulder blades drawing down their back, and heart center open as they fold forward. Most students will tend to shift their hips back while folding forward in order to maintain their balance and keep from falling forward. Encourage them to work on gradually keeping their legs vertical while folding forward by bringing their weight forward into the balls of their feet while keeping their heels firmly rooted down.

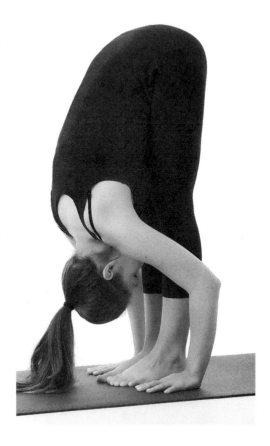

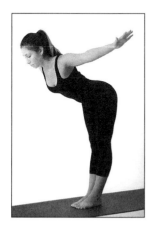

- Arm/Shoulder Option 1: "Swan-diving" is the easiest on the lower back and hamstrings, helps to maintain expansiveness across the heart center, and helps to open the shoulder girdle. This method can be contraindicated for students with unstable shoulders.

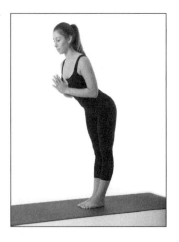

• Arm/Shoulder Option 2: Folding forward and down with the palms drawing through the center—through *anjali mudra*—can foster a sense of heart-centered awareness. It is relatively easy on the lower back and hamstrings, but the chest tends to collapse.

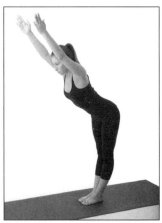

• Arm/Shoulder Option 3: Folding forward and down with the arms fully extended overhead, this option requires considerable lower back, leg, and core strength. If lacking strength in these areas, this method of folding can strain the lower back and hamstrings.

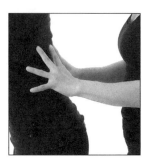

Use Finger Spreads to cue lifting the ribs away from the hips.

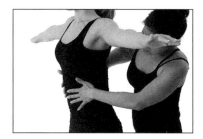

Use Light Touch to cue the floating ribs from protruding out.

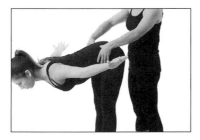

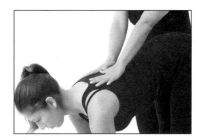

Use Hip Handles with Clasping Rotation to encourage maximum comfortable forward rotation of the pelvis as the primary source of the forward fold before placing the hands on the floor, blocks, or a wall.

While verbally cueing students to draw the spine long and sternum forward in the halfway-up position, use Opposite Rotation at the shoulder blades to cue the shoulder blades down the back and the sternum away from the belly, before cueing to fold farther down.

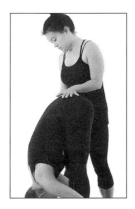

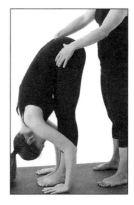

Use an Open Palm on the top of the sacrum to cue alignment of the hips over the ankles.

Use Hip Handles with Clasping Rotation to ground the legs and posteriorly rotate the pelvis as the student inhales to transition up from the forward fold, thereby easing pressure in the lower back.

Modification

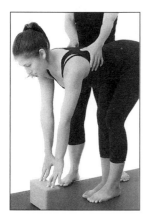

If the student is unable to fold forward halfway without rounding the spine, offer blocks to place under the hands on the floor and suggest bending the knees to take it easier on the lower back and hamstrings.

Explore Further

Teaching Yoga: page 160

Yoga Sequencing: page 444

Teaching Yoga Resource Center: www.markstephensyoga.com/resources

Padangusthasana (Big Toe Pose)

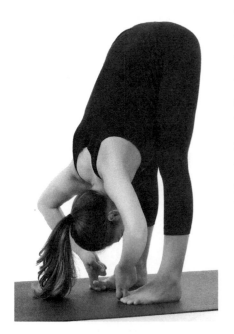

With pada bandha in both feet, for Padangusthasana, fold forward as for Uttanasana, then clasp and pull up on the big toes while stretching the chest forward as for Ardha Uttanasana; then fold down, stretching the elbows away from each other and shrugging the shoulder blades down the back. Start as for Uttanasana. Radiate down through the legs to ground the feet firmly and activate the legs; internally rotate the femurs, pitch the pubic bone back and up, and stretch the sternum toward the floor. Try to bring the weight forward while grounding the heels. Lengthen the spine from the strength and action in the legs.

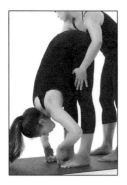

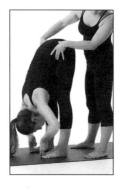

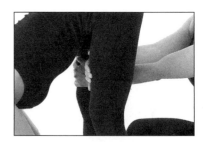

Use a light Finger Draw above the knees to clarify or awaken engagement of the quadriceps muscles.

Use Hip Handles to cue maximum anterior rotation of the pelvis and to cue centering of the pelvis over the feet (sitting bones above the heels).

Use Crossed Wrists to cue internal rotation of the thighs.

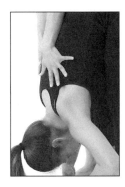

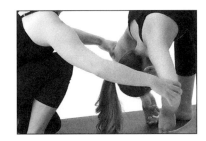

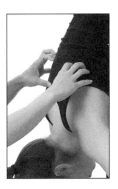

With Open Palms placed wide across the shoulder blades, adduct the hands, giving an Opposite Rotation cue: thumbs cue the medial scapulae down the back while fingers cue extension of the sternum away from the belly.

Use Light Hands to cue elbows away from each other and in line with the wrists and shoulders.

If the shoulders are shrugged toward the neck, use a light Finger Draw to cue the shoulder blades down against the back ribs.

Modification

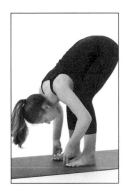

If unable to clasp the big toes with straight legs, keep the knees bent.

Variation

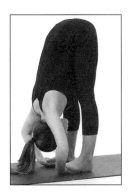

For wrist therapy and a deeper forward bend, offer Pada Hastasana (Hand to Foot Pose).

Explore Further

Teaching Yoga: page 184

Yoga Sequencing: page 403

Teaching Yoga Resource Center:
   www.markstephensyoga.com/resources

Malasana (Garland Pose)

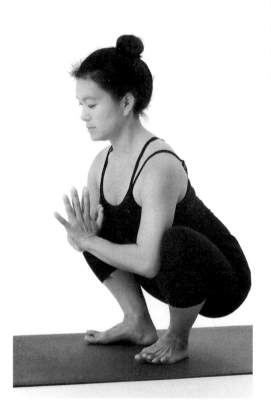

From Tadasana, verbally cue and demonstrate separating the feet slightly wider than hip distance and then slowly bending the knees until in a fully squatted position (if necessary, do this against a wall or with use of a chair or block).

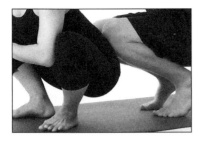

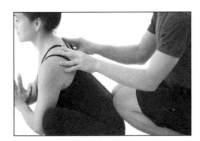

In Low Chair Stance, place your knees just above the upper rim of the student's pelvis to assist him or her in sitting stably and comfortably on the feet.

Draw Light Hands from the student's shoulders down the back while verbally cueing to lift the sternum.

Modification

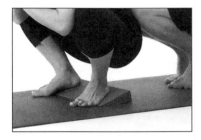

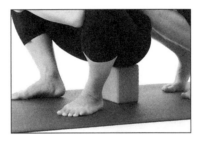

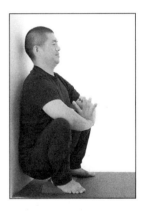

If the student is unable to root the heels into the floor, offer a rolled mat or wedge to place under the heels.

If the rolled mat or wedge prop is not adequate to support the student on the feet, offer a block (or two or more) to place under the sitting bones.

Students still having difficulty sitting up can practice this asana with the back against a wall.

Explore Further

Teaching Yoga: pages 327-29

Yoga Sequencing: page 397

Teaching Yoga Resource Center:
www.markstephensyoga.com/resources

Prasarita Padottanasana A (Spread-Leg Forward Fold Pose A)

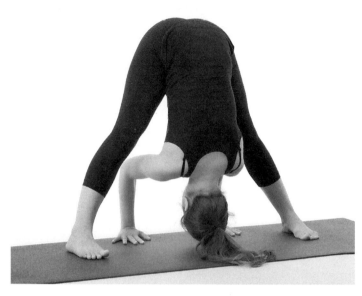

Start with the feet separated the length of one leg, outer edges of the feet parallel. The knees can be bent to relieve the hamstrings and the lower back. Slide the wrists back under the elbows and create the feeling of sliding the hands forward to lengthen the spine, drawing the shoulder blades down against the back ribs. The legs are straight and strong; slight internal rotation of the femurs eases anterior rotation of the pelvis, drawing the pubic bone back and up while stretching the belly button and sternum toward the floor. Try to bring the weight forward into the balls of the feet while grounding the fronts of the heels, hips directly over the heels; relax the neck.

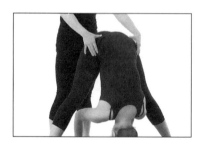

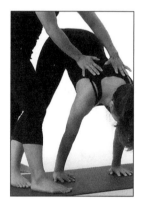

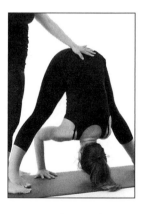

Use Hip Handles with Clasping Rotation to encourage maximum comfortable forward rotation of the pelvis as the primary source of the forward fold before folding through the torso and releasing the top of the head toward the floor.

While verbally cueing students to draw the spine long and sternum forward in the halfway-up position, use Opposite Rotation at the shoulder blades to cue the shoulder blades down the back and the sternum away from the belly, before cueing to fold farther down.

Use an Open Palm on the top of the sacrum to cue alignment of the hips over the ankles.

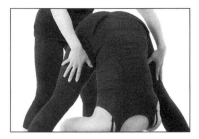

Use Light Touch of the fingers to clarify and suggest contraction of the quadriceps muscles.

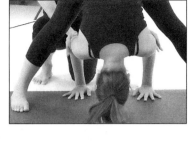

Use Light Touch of the fingers of Open Palms to cue alignment of the elbows with the shoulders.

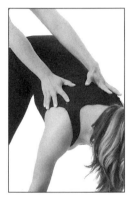

Preparing to come up, while verbally cueing students to draw the spine long and sternum forward in the halfway up position, use Opposite Rotation at the shoulder blades to cue the shoulder blades down the back and the sternum away from the belly, before cueing the transition to standing upright.

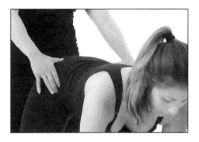

Use Hip Handles with Clasping Rotation to ground the legs and posteriorly rotate the pelvis as the student inhales to transition up from the forward fold, thereby easing pressure in the lower back.

Modification

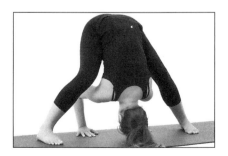

Keep the knees slightly bent to take it easier on the hamstrings and lower back.

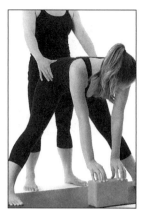

Place the hands on a block and lift the sternum forward while rotating the pelvis fully forward without folding the spine to take it easier on the lower back.

Explore Further

Teaching Yoga: page 180

Yoga Sequencing: page 416

Teaching Yoga Resource Center:
   www.markstephensyoga.com/resources

Prasarita Padottanasana C (Spread-Leg Forward Fold Pose C)

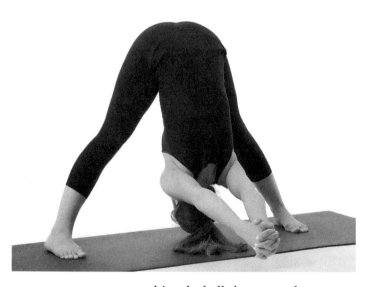

Start with the feet separated the length of one leg, outer edges of the feet parallel. The knees can be bent to relieve the hamstrings and lower back. Keep the shoulder blades rooted down against the back ribs while stretching the arm overhead and expanding across the chest (if the shoulders are tight, use a strap between the hands). The legs are straight and strong; slight internal rotation of the femurs eases anterior rotation of the pelvis, drawing the pubic bone back and up while stretching the belly button and sternum toward the floor. Try to bring the weight forward into the balls of the feet while grounding the fronts of the heels, hips directly over the heels; relax the neck.

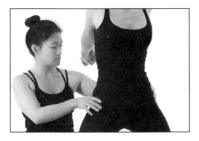

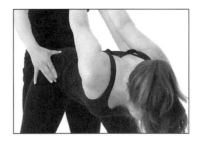

Use Hip handles to cue pelvic neutrality while verbally cueing the neutral extension of the spine (keep the floating ribs from protruding out as the student claps the hands behind the back).

Use Hip Handles with Clasping Rotation to encourage maximum comfortable forward rotation of the pelvis as the primary source of the forward fold before folding through the torso and releasing the top of the head toward the floor.

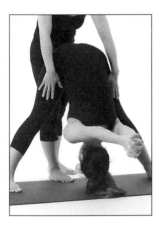

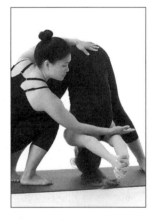

Use Light Touch of the fingers to clarify and suggest contraction of the quadriceps muscles.

Place an Open Palm on the top of the sacrum to stabilize positioning while placing the opposite forearm and hand across the student's upper arm to encourage additional shoulder extension. (A knee can also be braced behind the student's leg for added stability).

Modification

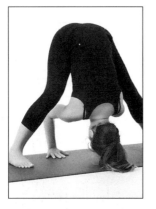

Keep the knees slightly bent to take it easier on the hamstrings and lower back.

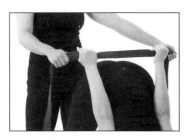

If the student is unable or barely able to clasp the hands behind the back, or if the arms will not lift more than a few inches away from the back, offer a strap to clasp with the hands shoulder distance apart (or wider for students with very tight shoulders).

Explore Further

Teaching Yoga: page 180

Yoga Sequencing: page 418

Teaching Yoga Resource Center:
   www.markstephensyoga.com/resources

Anjaneyasana (Low Lunge Pose)

In stepping the right foot back and releasing the knee to the floor for Anjaneyasana, emphasize maintaining the length of the spine and openness of the heart center. Students whose knees are sensitive to pressure when placed on the floor can place padding under the grounded knee. Consider offering students the following instructions to help break down and integrate the various actions in this asana: partially straighten the front leg, place the hands on the hips, and create a slight posterior pelvic tilt to find pelvic neutrality. Slowly bend the front knee to deepen the lunge and the stretch of the hip flexors while continuing to cultivate pelvic neutrality. Play with slowly moving in and out of the full depth of the lunge, gradually releasing into a deeper stretch in the hips and groin.

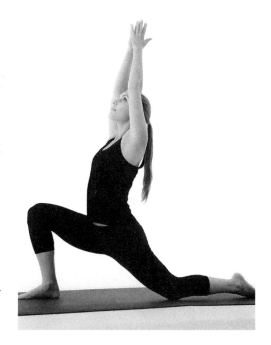

Once fully into the lunge, ask students to release their arms down by their sides, turn their palms out to externally rotate their arms, and then reach their arms overhead. With their arms overhead, ask students to look down for a moment and lightly soften their lower front ribs inward while maintaining pelvic neutrality, then try to reach their arms farther back without letting their lower front ribs protrude out. The arms can be held shoulder distance apart, and the head is held level. Invite students who can keep their elbows straight to press their palms together overhead while lifting through their sides, chest, back, arms, and fingertips. If it is okay with the neck, gaze at the thumbs.

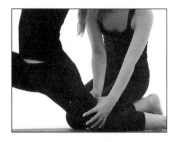

Use Light Hand or Clasping Rotation to cue internal rotation of the back thigh. Also cue the back foot to point straight back and press into the floor. Pad the knee if it's uncomfortable rooting it down.

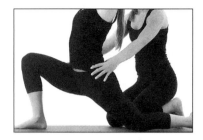

Use Hip Handles to cue pelvic neutrality. Note that most students anteriorly rotate the pelvis, especially as they deepen the lunge, bringing potentially stressful pressure to intervertebral disks in the lower back.

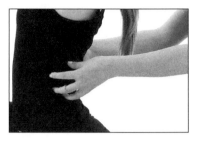

Use Finger Spreads to cue lengthening through the lower back and sides.

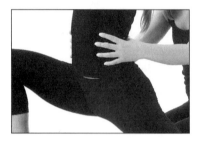

Use Light Hand on the lower side ribs to cue neutral spinal extension (against the tendency to arch the back).

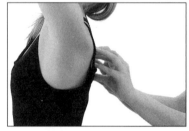

Use Finger Draws to cue the shoulder blades down the back.

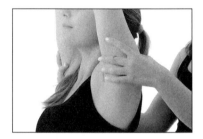

Use Clasping Rotation to cue external rotation and flexion of the arms.

Explore Further

Teaching Yoga: page 162

Yoga Sequencing: page 364

Teaching Yoga Resource Center:
www.markstephensyoga.com/resources

Ashta Chandrasana (Crescent Pose or High Lunge Pose)

From Tadasana, instruct students to step their left foot back about four feet, or alternatively, from Adho Mukha Svanasana, ask students to step their right foot forward next to their right hand, and then draw their hands to their hips while pressing the front leg straight. Cue students to use their hands to position the pelvis level while pressing back strongly through the lifted back heel, then to keep the pelvis level and the back leg engaged while bending the front knee straight forward into alignment above (not beyond) the heel. Alternately extending and flexing the front knee allows easier release of the hip flexors. Next, cue students to release their arms down by their sides, turn the palms out to externally rotate the arms, then reach the arms out and up overhead, either shoulder distance apart or, if they can keep their elbows fully extended, to press the palms together while gazing either forward or to the thumb tips.

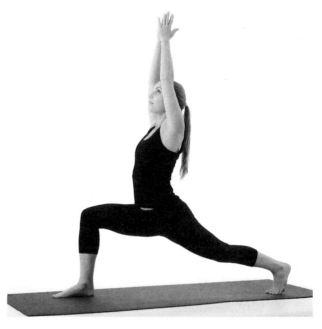

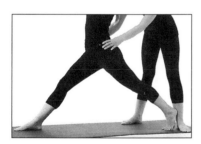

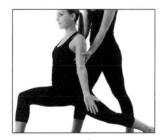

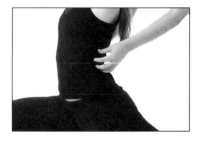

With your foot placed against the student's back heel and your hands placed for Hip Handles, cue the student to slowly bend the front knee while pressing the back heel into your foot, using the Hip Handles to keep the student's pelvis from rotating forward.

As you cue the student to release the arms down by the sides, use Clasping Rotation on the upper arms to cue their external rotation as you verbally cue the student to extend the arms out and up overhead.

Use Finger Spreads to cue the student to lift the lower rim of the rib cage up away from the upper rim of the hips, thereby creating more length through the lower back.

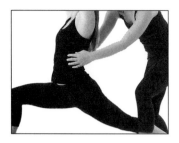

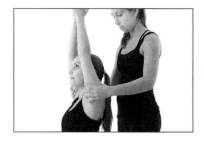

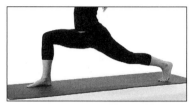

Use Light Hands and Open Palms to cue the student to keep the floating ribs from protruding out, thereby minimizing the arch of the spine while encouraging its elongation.

While verbally cueing the student to stretch the arms overhead, encourage him or her to root the upper arms down and into the shoulder socket, using Clasping Rotation at the upper arms to cue this action.

If the student's front knee is beyond the heel (out over or even beyond the foot), cue the student to wiggle the back foot back until the front knee in aligned over the heel.

Modification

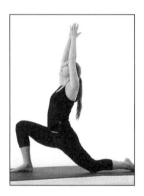

If Ashta Chandrasana is too intense or if there is tension in the front knee, cue the student to practice Anjaneyasana instead.

Explore Further

Teaching Yoga: pages 172–73

Yoga Sequencing: pages 368–69

Teaching Yoga Resource Center:
www.markstephensyoga.com/resources

Utthita Trikonasana (Extended Triangle Pose)

Start with the feet separated the length of one leg; turn the right foot out ninety degrees, and the left slightly in. Shift the hips to the left, pressing the right sitting bone toward the left while reaching out to the right through the spine and arm to the point of maximum extension, then release the hand onto the lower leg or ankle. Offer the option of looking down to make it easier on the neck. Suggest initially bringing the hand higher up the shin to ease the lengthening and slight rotation of the spine. The legs are straight and strong without hyperextending the knees; the front leg's kneecap is lifted and pointed forward; lateral flexion of the spine is minimized; the torso is turned to the side wall and aligned directly over the leg. The neck long, radiate out from heart center through both arms and fingertips.

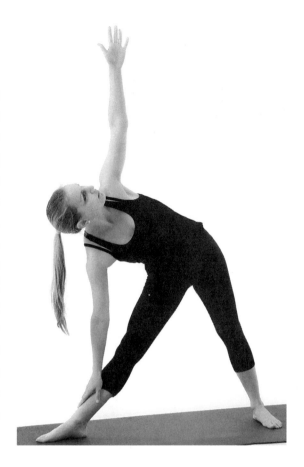

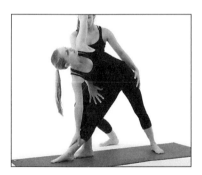

Standing next to the student in Hip Stance positioning, use your hip to cue pressing the hip of the front leg toward the back foot while using Open Palms positioning to cue the back leg back (opening the hips) and to cue the front knee to point forward.

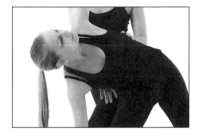

Standing next to the student in Hip Stance, use Opposite Rotation to cue elongation and rotation of the torso, cueing the lower ribs forward and under, the upper ribs back and down.

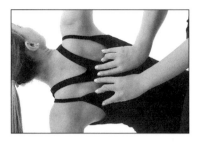

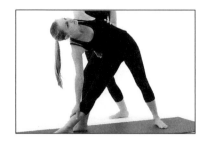

Use Finger Draws to cue the shoulder blades down against the back ribs while verbally cueing the student to radiate out from the sternum through the fingers.

If the student is slumping forward or laterally arching the mid-spine, cue drawing the lower hand higher up the shin (or onto a chair or block).

Modification

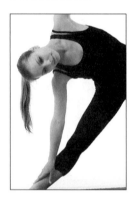

If it troubles the neck holding the head up, relax the neck and ease the head down, and gaze down.

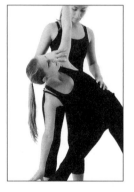

If the student is slumping forward or laterally arching the mid-spine, cue drawing the lower hand higher up the shin (or onto a chair or block), then stand behind the back and cue the student to draw the back against you and into alignment over the front leg.

Explore Further

Teaching Yoga: page 178

Yoga Sequencing: page 447

Teaching Yoga Resource Center: www.markstephensyoga.com/resources

---

Utthita Parsvakonasana (Extended Side Angle Pose)

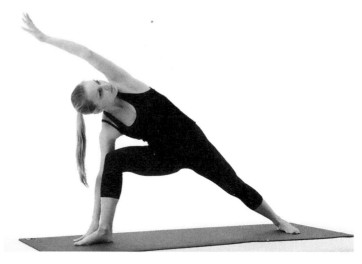

From Virabhadrasana II (Warrior II Pose), keep the feet grounded and reach out through the right arm and side, initially placing the elbow on the knee; drawing the shoulder blades down the back, revolve the torso open, reach the left arm down the back leg, turn the palm up to feel external rotation of the arm, then reach the arm overhead; over time, bring the lower fingertips or palm to a block or the floor to the inside of the front foot, and over time to the outside of the foot. Minimize lateral flexion of the spine while rotating the torso open; maintain a strong line of energy from grounded back foot through the extended fingertips; press the elbow or shoulder against the knee isometrically to keep the knee aligned and leverage rotation of the torso; gaze to the upper fingertips or relax the neck and look across the room or to the floor.

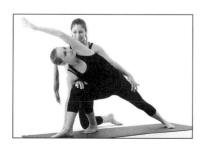

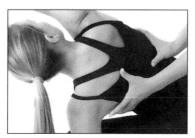

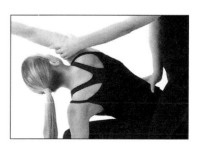

In One Knee Down Stance, use Hip-to-Hip positioning to stabilize the student's front hip position while using Open Palms in the front knee and back thigh to cue alignment of the front knee and opening across the front of the pelvis.

Standing next to the student, use Opposite Open Palms to cue elongation and rotation of the torso, cueing the lower ribs forward and under, the upper ribs back and down.

Use Clasping Rotation on the upper arm to cue its external rotation.

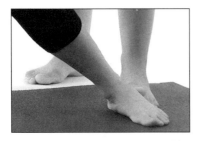

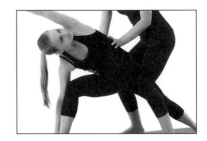

Place a toe on the student's back heel to cue its active grounding while leaning forward to use Opposite Open Palms to cue elongation and rotation of the torso, cueing the lower ribs forward and under, the upper ribs back and down.

In a slightly wide and scissored Mountain Stance, use the knees to press equally against the back thigh and the front hip to cue their alignment and energetic actions while using your hands for torso and arm cues, as described above.

Modification

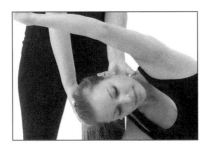

If it troubles the neck holding the head up, relax the neck and ease the head down, and gaze down.

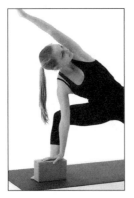

If unable to keep the spine fully elongated and the torso toward ninety degrees away from the floor (facing the side of the room), place the lower hand on a block to the inside of the front foot, or place that elbow on the front knee.

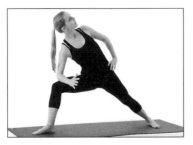

If in the basic modified position the student is unable draw the arm overhead, suggest placing that hand on the upper hip and focusing on lengthening the spine and twisting open.

Variation

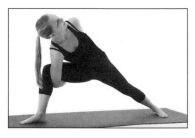

Wrap the lower arm under the lower leg and draw the upper arm behind the back to clasp that wrist, and straighten that arm while using that clasp next to the hip to press that hip under and leverage the twist of the torso.

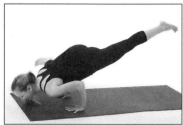

If wrapped and clasped, explore transitioning to Eka Pada Koundinyasana A (One-Leg Sage Koundinya's Pose A) and Astavakrasana (Eight-Angle Pose) on the way to Chaturanga Dandasana (Four-Limbed Staff Pose).

Explore Further

Teaching Yoga: page 177

Yoga Sequencing: page 446

Teaching Yoga Resource Center: www.markstephensyoga.com/resources

Ardha Chandrasana (Half Moon Pose)

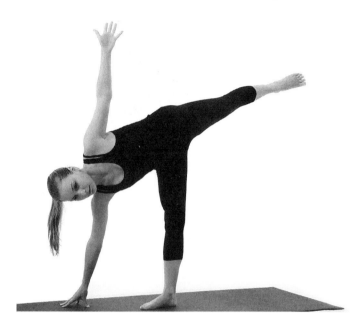

Transition in stages from Utthita Trikonasana by bending the front knee, placing the fingertips about a foot in from the front foot (on the floor or on a block), sliding the back foot closer to the front foot until fully weighting the front foot and hand, then slowly beginning to straighten the front leg while keeping the back hip rotated fully open. Maintain external rotation of the hips while transitioning; keep the standing foot from turning in; extend the lifted leg straight back from the hip; radiate out from the belly through the legs and spine, and from the heart center radiate out through the fingertips.

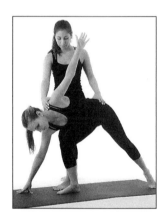

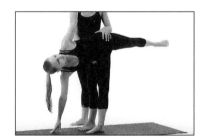

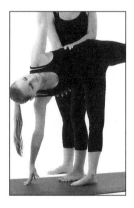

From Trikonasana, use Hip Stance with Open Palm at the shoulder and move with the student to stabilize and ease the transition forward onto one foot, verbally cueing to keep the foot from turning in.

Maintain or come into Hip Stance to assist balance and use Open Palms to cue maintaining the open rotation of the pelvis.

Use Opposite Open Palms to cue elongation and rotation of the torso, cueing the lower ribs forward and under, the upper ribs back and down.

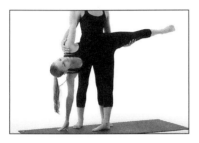

Use Open Palms to lightly cue alignment of the lifted leg straight back from the hip and the upper shoulder back to position the student as though against a wall.

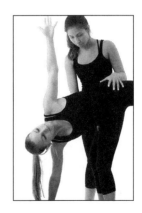

Maintain or come into Hip Stance to assist balance in transitioning back into Trikonasana.

Modification

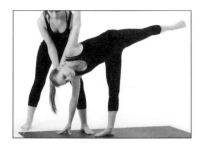

If it troubles the neck holding the head up, relax the neck and ease the head down, and gaze down.

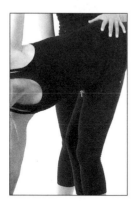

If the knee of the standing leg is shaking, do not press it straight, and either release out of the asana or bend the knee.

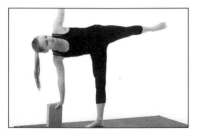

If unable to fully turn the torso to face the side of the room, place the fingertips of the lower hand high on a block.

Variation

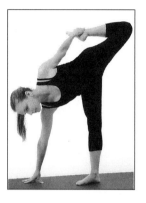

If fully open and stable in the basic asana, explore bending the lifted knee to bring that foot behind the back to clasp it with the upper hand, and if possible position the hand on top of the foot as for Bhekasana (Frog Pose) and press that foot in toward the outer hip. Do not bring the knee forward to get the clasp, as this will cause that hip to rotate forward, bringing excessive pressure into that hip joint.

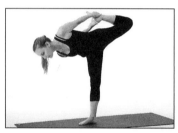

If in easy and stable balance, lift the lower hand off the floor and clasp the foot with both hands.

Explore Further

Teaching Yoga: page 178

Yoga Sequencing: page 366

Teaching Yoga Resource Center:
www.markstephensyoga.com/resources

Parsvottanasana (Intense Extended Side Stretch Pose)

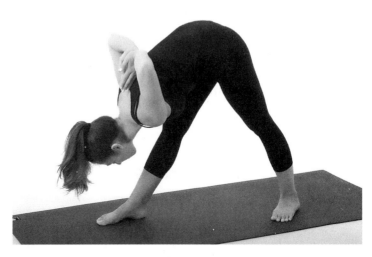

Start with a Prasarita stance, initially with the feet separated the length of one leg, then bring the feet a few inches closer together. With the hands on the hips, turn the right foot out ninety degrees, then lift and replace the left foot on the floor, positioning it more or less parallel to the right, as much or as little as it takes to square the hips toward the front of the mat while still feeling a stretch in the left groin. Place the palms together behind the back in reverse prayer position (or clasp wrists or elbows); keep both legs straight and strong; keep the hips even and level by pressing down through the right leg and foot, drawing the right hip back, and rooting the back heel firmly down, internally rotating the thigh of the back leg. Rooting through the legs and feet, lift through the spine, opening across the heart center, then slowly rotate the pelvis anteriorly, the public bone drawing back and up, while stretching the belly button toward the thigh and the sternum toward the toes.

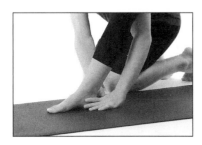

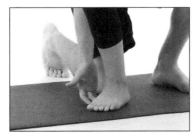

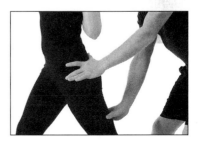

Cue the front foot to point straight forward and either in alignment with the back of the back heel or a wider lateral stance for easier alignment of the hips and easier lateral balance.

Highlight pada bandha in the back foot to help keep it level, balanced in its rooting, and grounded, and to more easily internally rotate the thigh of that leg.

Using Open Palms, place one hand above the hip and one on the inner thigh to encourage internal rotation of the thigh as the source of the hip of the back leg moving forward.

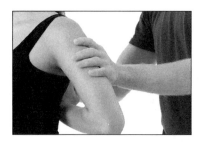 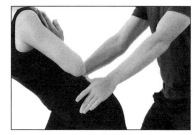 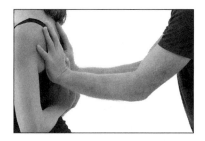

Instructing the student to abduct the arms to ninety degrees, use Clasping Rotation on the arms close to the shoulders to cue internal rotation of the arms, thereby easing positioning of the arms behind the back and palms together in reverse prayer position. Verbally cue (or use very light Open Palms) to cue the elbows back.

Verbally cueing the student to lift the chest slightly on each inhalation, using Open Palms placed wide across the shoulder blades, adduct the hands, giving an Opposite Rotation cue: thumbs cue the medial scapulae down the back while fingers cue extension of the sternum away from the belly.

Use Hip Handles with Clasping Rotation to encourage maximum comfortable forward rotation of the pelvis as the primary source of the forward fold before folding through the torso in bringing the sternum toward the toes.

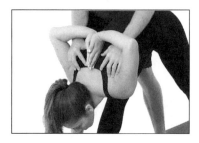 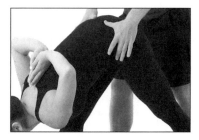

On each exhalation, verbally cue to maintain the greater length of the sternum away from the belly while folding farther forward and down, using Finger Draws on the back to add emphasis.

Use Hip Handles with Clasping Rotation to ground the legs and posteriorly rotate the pelvis as the student inhales to transition up from the forward fold, thereby easing pressure in the lower back.

Modification

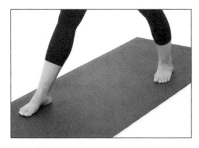

Turning the back foot in slightly less than the traditional sixty degrees or taking a slightly wider lateral stance will ease alignment of the legs, hips, and pelvis.

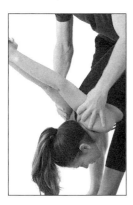

If unable to position the hands in reverse prayer, clasp the elbows.

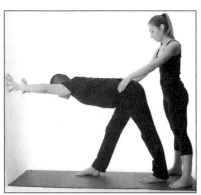

Practice with the hands on a wall, chair, or blocks to more easily explore the actions of the feet, legs, and pelvis, and to explore without straining the hamstrings or lower back.

Variation

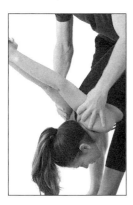

Interlace the fingers behind the back and stretch the arms overhead without collapsing the spine.

Explore Further

Teaching Yoga: page 181

Yoga Sequencing: page 412

Teaching Yoga Resource Center:
   www.markstephensyoga.com/resources

Parivrtta Trikonasana (Revolved Triangle Pose)

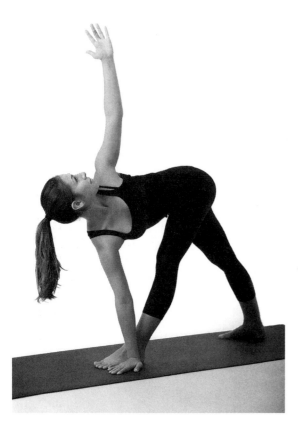

Most students will shift their hips in an attempt to bring their hand to the floor or to turn their torso farther to the right, which tends to bring the twist more into the lower back rather than into the thoracic spine; encourage students to make the stable positioning of their hips and legs more interesting than placement of their hand or rotation of their torso. Start with the left fingertips high on a block (or a wall or chair), and the right hand on the hip to encourage the hip back and the torso to revolve open. In extending the right arm up, remind students to keep that arm from going back beyond the plane of their shoulders. If the neck is strained, drop the head. The legs and hips are identical to the upright starting position for Parsvottanasana. With the right leg forward, bring the right hand to the right hip to keep the hip positioned there, and reach the left arm up and rotate the pelvis forward, bringing the right hand to the floor (or a block or chair) to the inside (over time to the outside) of the right foot, rotating the torso open to the right while maintaining the positioning of the legs and hips. Draw the shoulder blades down the back and radiate out from the heart center through the arms and fingertips.

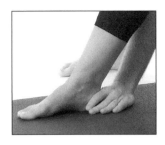

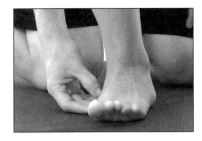

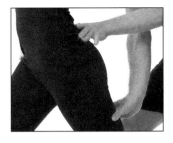

Cue the front foot to point straight forward and either in alignment with the back of the back heel or a wider lateral stance for easier alignment of the hips and easier lateral balance.

Highlight pada bandha in the back foot to help keep it level, balanced in its rooting, and grounded, and to more easily internally rotate the thigh of that leg. Turning that foot in slightly less than the traditional sixty degrees will ease alignment of the legs, hips, and pelvis.

Using Open Palms, place one hand above the hip and one on the inner thigh to encourage internal rotation of the thigh as the source of the hip of the back leg moving forward.

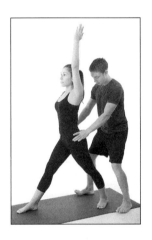

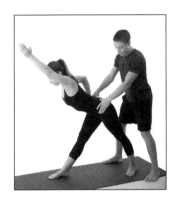

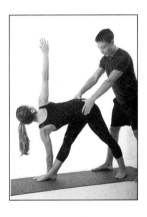

First using Hip Handles with Clasping Rotation to cue pelvis neutrality in relation to the spine, instruct stretching the lifted arm straight up to lengthen through that side both in the preparatory position and in the next step.

Use Hip Handles with Clasping Rotation to encourage maximum comfortable forward rotation of the pelvis as the primary source of the forward fold before verbally cueing placement of the hand on a block or the floor.

Using Hip Handles to align and stabilize the pelvis, verbally cue the student to rotate through the mid-torso while extending the upper arm straight up.

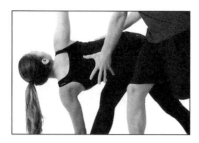
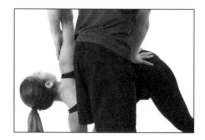

Standing the same direction as the student with Hip-to-Hip placement to stabilize balance, use Open Palms on each side of the torso to encourage lengthening and rotation of the torso by cueing the lower ribs forward and under, the upper ribs back and down.

Standing the opposite direction of the student with Hip-to-Hip placement to stabilize balance, use an Open Palm on the pelvis to steer the pelvis level and on the upper shoulder to encourage the torso to rotate.

Modification

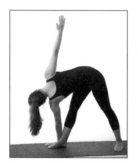

If it troubles the neck holding the head up, relax the neck and ease the head down and gaze down.

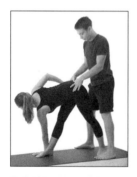

If unable to twist the torso to where the shoulders are turned ninety degrees to the floor without shifting from the level position of the pelvis, cue placing the lifted hand on that hip to press it back, help elongate the spine, and encourage the twist.

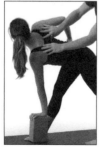

To more easily lengthen the spine and twist the torso, place the hand on a block.

Explore Further

Teaching Yoga: page 181

Yoga Sequencing: page 409

Teaching Yoga Resource Center:
    www.markstephensyoga.com/resources

Parivrtta Parsvakonasana (Revolved Extended Side Angle Pose)

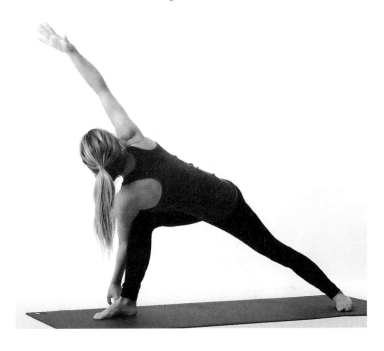

Start with the right foot forward in Ashta Chandrasana, or more challengingly, in Virabhadrasana I. Place the left hand on the left hip to help stabilize the hip in that position. Emphasize the importance of this positioning and the alignment of the front knee over the heel. Reach the right arm straight up to help lengthen through the right side of the torso, then stretch forward while twisting to the left, placing the left elbow on the right knee for a prayer positioning, or, if students have greater rotational flexibility and open hips, draw the shoulder across the knee and the hand to the floor outside the left foot. Finally, stretch the left arm overhead, externally rotating the arm while rotating the torso to the left. Emphasize alignment of the front knee above the front heel and the left hip directly back from that knee as in Virabhadrasana I. Keeping the back heel lifted in the Ashta Chandrasana positioning offers a more accessible preparatory approach. Keep the back leg strongly engaged. If in the full form of the asana with the back heel down, commit to rooting the outer edge of that foot to help rotate that hip forward.

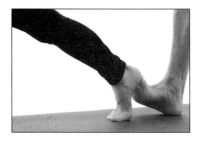

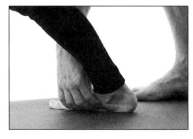

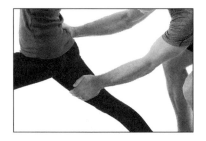

For the more accessible Ashta Chandrasana option, ask the student to keep the back heel lifted and place your foot to that heel to suggest energizing out through that leg and heel.

In the traditional Virabhadrasana I positioning with the back heel turned in and rooted down, highlight pada bandha in that foot to help keep it level, balanced in its grounding, and to more easily internally rotate the thigh of that leg.

Using Open Palms, place one hand above the hip and one on the inner thigh to encourage internal rotation of the thigh as the source of the hip of the back leg moving forward.

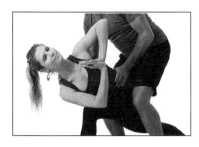

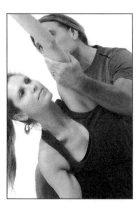

Depending on your relative height and that of the student, you can straddle the student and use Knee Bracing to stabilize the student's balance while using your hands for upper body cues.

Use Clasping Rotation to cue external rotation of the arm. Give this cue proximally—close to the shoulder and no more distal than a few inches above the elbow.

Modification

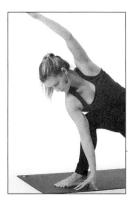

If it troubles the neck holding the head up, relax the neck and ease the head down, and gaze down.

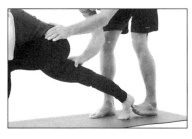

If unable to keep the front hip from lifting and splaying out and that knee from splaying in, instruct lifting and pressing the back heel straight back (Ashta Chandrasana positioning) while using Open Palms to cue internal rotation of the back thigh and rotation of that hip forward. Use all other cues given for the pelvis, torso, and arm.

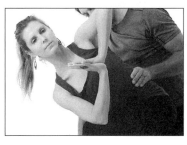

If unable to draw the shoulder across the knee without losing alignment of the leg or collapsing the spine and chest, instruct a prayer twist, and with Open Palms placed on each side of the torso, encourage lengthening and rotation of the torso by cueing the lower ribs forward and under, the upper ribs back and down.

Variation

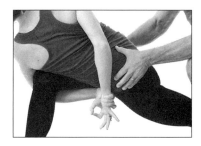

If full expression of the asana is easily accessible, instruct wrapping and clasping the wrists of the upper arm behind the back. This variation is perfectly self-adjusting, but cue to highlight the tendency to lose proper rooting of the back foot and alignment of the hips, front knee, and spine.

Virabhadrasana I (Warrior I Pose)

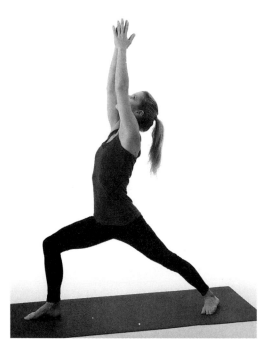

In transitioning from Adho Mukha Svanasana to Virabhadrasana I, there are two basic techniques. In traditional Ashtanga Vinyasa yoga, the left heel is turned in about halfway and rooted down before stepping the right foot forward. In many Vinyasa Flow classes, the right leg is first extended back and up while inhaling, then when exhaling, the foot is drawn forward and placed next to the right hand. When using either method, consider first instructing Ashta Chandrasana rather than Virabhadrasana I as a way of introducing high lunge poses and offering the space in which to gently release through the hip flexors and groin while ensuring that students understand the important alignment principle of knee-over-heel. In further preparation for either the first Ashta Chandrasana or Virabhadrasana I, ask students to come high onto their fingertips, draw their shoulder blades down their back, and extend the sternum forward to draw more length through the spine and create more space around the neck.

In either Ashta Chandrasana or Virabhadrasana I, ask students to initially straighten their front leg all the way while drawing their torso all the way up into a vertical position, place their hands on their hips, and bring the pelvis to a place of neutrality while pressing the back leg straight and strong. If starting with Ashta Chandrasana, next cue students to draw their back heel in and down to the floor to establish the foundation there for Virabhadrasana I: cultivate pada bandha, rotate the back hip forward, the inner thigh of the back leg rotating back and the pelvis level. With the hands still on the hips, ask students to try to maintain as much pelvic neutrality as they can—space between their hip and front thigh—while slowing bending their front leg and consciously guiding their knee toward the little-toe side of the foot. It is very important to ensure that the front knee does not travel out beyond the heel; allowing the knee to go farther forward places excessive pressure on the ACL. If a student feels pressure in the back knee or lower back when bending the front knee into Virabhadrasana I, guide that person to back out of the lunge or explore bending the knee less deeply. Keeping the back heel lifted straight up in the Ashta Chandrasana positioning will also reduce or eliminate the pressure in the back knee and lower back.

In either asana, once students are up in the lunge position, ask them to release their arms down by their sides, turn their palms out to feel the external rotation of their arms at the shoulder joint, and then reach their arms out and up overhead while keeping the shoulder blades rooted down and in against their back ribs. Cue the class to look down for a moment and draw their lower front ribs slightly in, then try to maintain that positioning while bringing the gaze forward and the arms back. This will help students to develop neutral extension of the spine with greater shoulder flexion, which is intrinsically beneficial and helpful in creating the body intelligence for asanas such as Adho Mukha Vrksasana (Handstand). Encourage students who can keep their arms straight to draw their palms together overhead, and if it is okay with the neck, to gaze up to the tips of their thumbs.

To deepen the experience of Virabhadrasana I, emphasize the steady grounding of the feet, internal rotation of the back leg while pressing the shin firmly back to further ground the back heel, pada bandha in both feet, mula bandha, and steady energetic lifting through the spine, through the heart center, and out through the fingertips. Suggest lifting the lower rim of the ribs up and away from the upper rims of the hips to create more space and ease in the lower back. The breath should be steady and even, the eyes soft, the heart open. Virabhadrasana I is an excellent asana in which to teach multiple lines of energy, the relationship between roots and extension, and the balance of sthira and sukham. In the transition from Virabhadrasana I to Chaturanga Dandasana (Four-Limbed Staff Pose), encourage students to keep the movement simple, fluid, and connected to the breath. You will observe many students, especially advancing beginners, keeping one foot off the floor all the way into and even through Chaturanga Dandasana. This undermines the stable foundation of Chaturanga Dandasana; the integrity of Four-Limbed Staff Pose is lost to an asymmetrical three-limb variation that compromises the balanced movement into Urdhva Mukha Svanasana (Upward-Facing Dog Pose). Done repetitively, this can destabilize the sacroiliac joint and lead to potentially chronic lower-back problems.

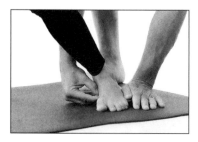

Use Finger Flicks and Open Palms to cue pada bandha in the back foot.

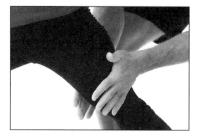

Place a toe on the student's back heel to cue its active grounding while using Open Palms to cue internal rotation of the back thigh as the source of that hip moving forward toward alignment with the other hip.

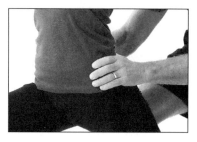

Use Hip Handles with Clasping Rotation to cue pelvic neutrality and to renew the effort to rotate the back hip forward, and use Hip Handles to cue the level and neutral positioning of the pelvis.

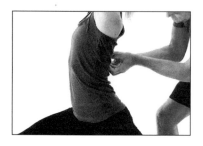

Use Finger Spreads to encourage lifting the rib cage evenly up and away from the pelvis.

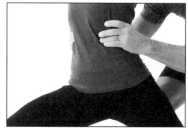

Use Open Palms to cue keeping the floating ribs from protruding out, thus helping cultivate neutral extension of the spine.

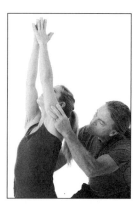

Use Clasping Rotation to cue and assist the lifting and external rotation of the arms.

Modification

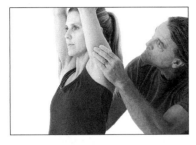

If it troubles the neck looking up, position the head level and gaze forward.

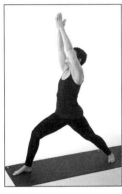

If a student reports discomfort in the lower back, cue straightening the front leg to the extent it takes to relieve that tension.

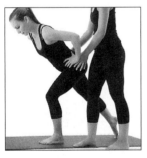

If a student reports sharp pain or tension in the back knee, cue lifting and pressing the back heel straight back to take the twisting effect away from the knee (thus coming into Ashta Chandrasana).

Explore Further

Teaching Yoga: page 172

Yoga Sequencing: page 450

Teaching Yoga Resource Center:
   www.markstephensyoga.com/resources

Virabhadrasana II (Warrior II Pose)

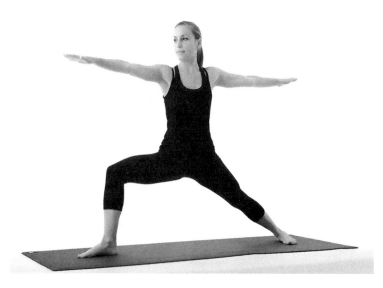

Start in a wide Prasarita stance, turning the right foot out, the left foot slightly in, slowly bending the right knee while guiding it toward the little-toe side of the foot; if the knee goes beyond the heel, crawl the toes farther forward for a longer stance. If starting from Virabhadrasana I, emphasize keeping front knee alignment while pressing the other thigh back. The front knee is aligned directly above the heel (it will tend to splay in); the front sitting bone draws under; hips are level, pelvis neutral, back leg firm with the arch lifted; shoulder blades are down the back; energy runs up through spine and out from the heart center through the fingertips. Press through the feet to release.

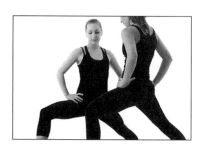

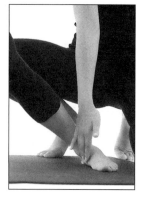

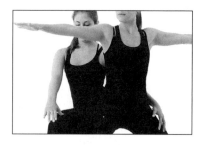

Mirroring a wide Prasarita stance, visually and verbally cue turning one foot out ninety degrees and the other foot slightly in, with front foot to back heel; level the hips with pelvic neutrality, and level the arms with the shoulder blades rooted down against the back ribs.

Visually and verbally cue bending the front knee into alignment directly above the knee; if it goes beyond the knee, cue crawling the toes forward to position the heel under the knee, then use Finger Flicks and Open Palms to cue pada bandha in the back foot.

In One Knee Down Stance, use Hip-to-Hip positioning to stabilize the student's front hip position while using Open Palms on the front knee and back thigh to cue alignment of the front knee and opening across the front of the pelvis.

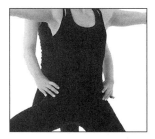

If the student's pelvis is rotated forward, verbally cue to partially straighten the front knee, then use Hip Handles with Clasping Rotation to cue pelvic neutrality while the student bends the knee into a deeper lunge.

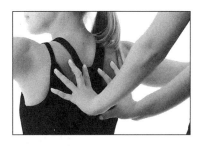

Use Finger Spreads to cue greater lengthening up through the spine.

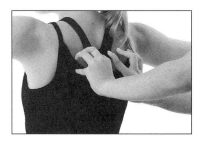

Use Finger draws at the shoulder blades or light Clasping Rotation at the tops of the shoulders to cue the shoulder blades down against the back ribs.

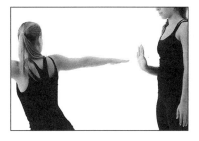

Use a hand for visual reference while saying "Reach into my hand" to cue the student to align the torso vertically (rather than out over the front leg).

Modification

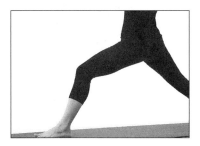

If in bending the knee it insists on splaying in and/or the pelvis insists on rotating forward, cue the student to bend the knee less far.

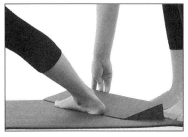

If the student reports strain or tension in the back ankle, offer a wedge to slightly elevate the outer edge of that foot.

Variation

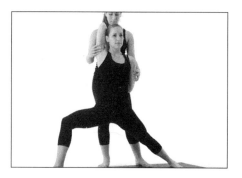

Explore various arm positions (Eagle or Cow Face arms) to focus on shoulder stretches related to where you are going with the overall sequence of asanas.

Explore Further

Teaching Yoga: page 177

Yoga Sequencing: page 451

Teaching Yoga Resource Center:
www.markstephensyoga.com/resources

Virabhadrasana III (Warrior III Pose)

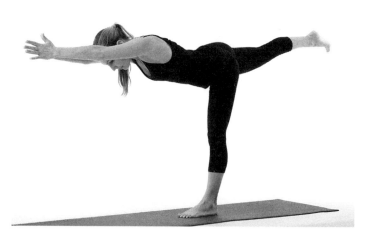

This asana is most easily learned with the hands on a wall. Explore transitioning into it from Ashta Chandrasana, springing lightly forward onto the front foot and leg and back into Ashta Chandrasana, eventually keeping the weight on the front foot and exploring the slow, steady straightening of the front leg while lifting the back leg eventually level with the hips; offer the option of having the arms back by the sides to make it easier on the lower back, or out like an airplane for easier balance. Do not lock the knee of the standing leg. Firm the thigh of the standing leg, keeping the ankle stable and the kneecap pointing forward; keep the hips level and internally rotate the femur of the lifted leg; lengthen through the side of the torso and chest; in the full asana, reach the arms forward, eventually pressing the palms together and gazing to the thumbs.

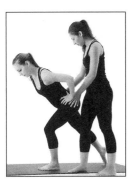

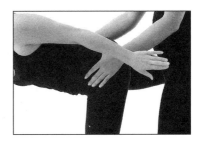

In transitioning from Ashta Chandrasana, cue level hips while assisting the transition onto one foot.

Stand on the standing leg side and use Hip Handles to cue the level alignment of the pelvis and to assist in stabilizing the student's balance.

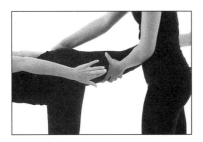

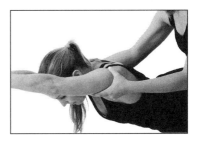

With Open Palms, use one hand to cue keeping the hips level and the other hand to cue extension and internal rotation of the lifted leg and extension of that knee.

Use Clasping Rotation to cue external rotation, flexion, and adduction of the arms.

Modification

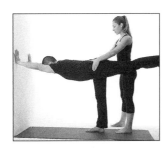

Practice at a wall with hands on the wall.

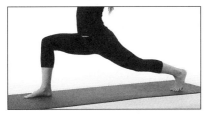

Keep the back foot on the floor.

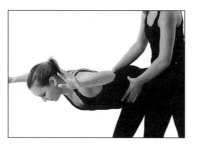

Keep the standing knee bent to take it easier on the knee and hip.

Explore Further

Teaching Yoga: page 182

Yoga Sequencing: page 452

Teaching Yoga Resource Center:
  www.markstephensyoga.com/resources

Parivrtta Ardha Chandrasana (Revolved Half Moon Pose)

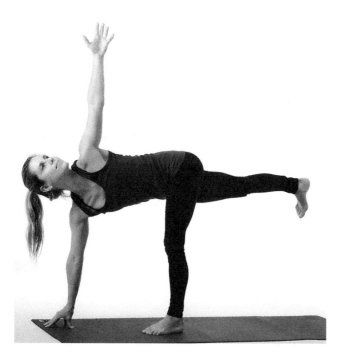

As with Parivrtta Trikonasana, many students tend to compromise the stable positioning of the legs and hips in order to create the feeling or appearance of a deeper twist; cue keeping the hips level and the back leg lifted and energized, then twist from there. The legs and hips are identical to their positioning in Virabhadrasana III. Standing on the right leg, bring the left hand (initially the fingertips) to a block or the floor directly under the left shoulder, and consider the option of placing the right hand on the right hip as offered in Parivrtta Trikonasana; rotating the torso to the right, eventually reach the right arm up.

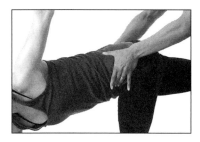 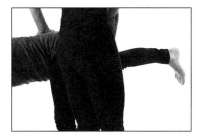 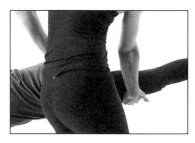

Use Light Hands to cue the pelvis level with the floor.

Stand on the student's standing-leg side facing the lifted leg with Hip Stance to stabilize balance.

Use Light Hands (if minimal indication) or Clasping Rotation (if greater indication) on the lifted leg to cue its full extension straight back from the hip and its internal rotation.

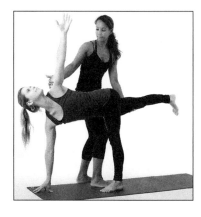

Using an Open Palm to cue keeping the lifted leg lifted toward level with the hip, use the other hand with Open Palm to cue at the shoulder for rotation of the torso.

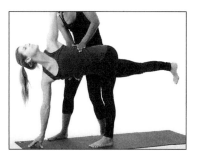

Explore turning the opposite direction with Hip Stance, and use Opposite Open Palms to cue elongation and rotation of the torso, cueing the lower ribs forward and under, the upper ribs back and down.

Modification

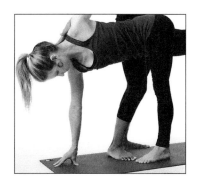

If it troubles the neck holding the head up, relax the neck and ease the head down, and gaze down.

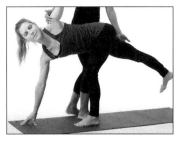

If it's too much on the hamstrings of the standing leg, keep that knee bent.

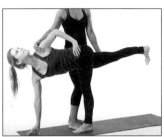

Consider the option of keeping the upper hand on the hip to press it back and encourage the twist rather than extending that arm up.

Variation

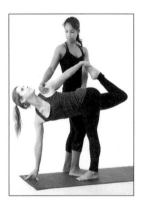

Explore reaching back with the upper hand to clasp the lifted foot, pulling that hand and foot away from each other to accentuate the twist while being very sensitive to the lower back.

Explore Further

Teaching Yoga: page 183

Yoga Sequencing: pages 405-6

Teaching Yoga Resource Center:
www.markstephensyoga.com/resources

Vrksasana (Tree Pose)

Start in Tadasana. Use the wall for support, heel of the lifted leg placed below the knee if unable to place it above. Keep the hands on the hips or at the heart; lightly cue even hips, pelvic neutrality, and abduction of the lifted leg. There is stability in the standing leg, the lifted heel above the knee, even hips, neutral pelvis, neutral spine, a steady gaze, and steady breath. Release slowly.

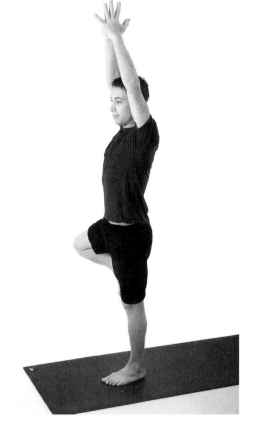

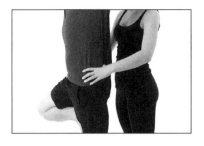

Use Hip Handles to lightly assist with balance and to cue level hips and pelvic neutrality.

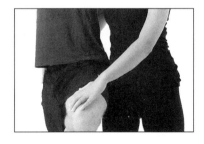

Use Hip-to-Hip Stance facing the direction of the student's lifted knee to stabilize the positioning of that hip while using an Open Palm to cue abduction of the lifted leg (try to keep the hip from moving back).

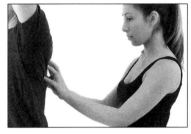

Use Finger Spreads to cue greater lengthening up through the spine.

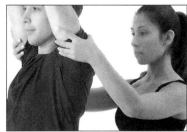

Use Clasping Rotation to cue external rotation, flexion, and adduction of the arms.

Modification

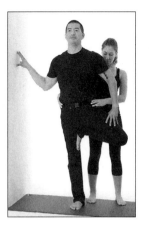

Use a wall for added support in exploring balance on one foot. If a student in unable to place the lifted foot entirely above the knee, cue to place it entirely below the knee, not against the knee at all.

Explore Further

Teaching Yoga: page 176

Yoga Sequencing: page 454

Teaching Yoga Resource Center:
  www.markstephensyoga.com/resources

Utthita Hasta Padangusthasana
(Extended Hand to Big Toe Pose)

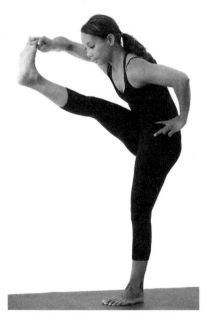

Start as for Utthita Hasta Padangusthasana A, then as with Vrksasana. Encourage students to be more interested in keeping their standing leg stable, hips level, and pelvis neutral than getting their lifted leg out to the side. Offer the option of using a strap around the foot of the lifted leg, or clasp that knee and keep it bent when abducting the thigh. Grounding down through the standing leg, feel more space through the standing hip, the spine, and out through the top of the head; expanding across the chest, explore looking over the shoulder to the opposite side of the lifted leg while extending that leg out on abduction. Breath and gaze are steady.

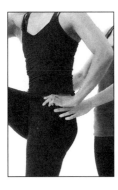

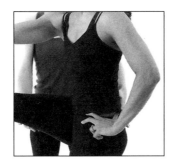

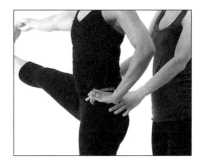

Standing behind the student, use Hip Handles with Clasping Rotation to cue and stabilize pelvic neutrality as the student lifts one leg.

Facing the student from the lifted leg side, use an Open Palm on the sacrum to cue pelvic neutrality while using Light Touch to cue lifting the lifted leg higher.

In the abducted B variation, use Hip Handles to cue keeping the hips level and even while the student moves the lifted leg to the side.

Modification

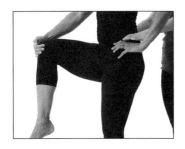

If unable to keep the standing leg straight and the spine tall, keep the knee of the lifted leg bent or place a strap around that foot.

Explore Further

Teaching Yoga: page 184

Yoga Sequencing: page 445

Teaching Yoga Resource Center:
www.markstephensyoga.com/resources

Parivrtta Hasta Padangusthasana
(Revolved Hand to Big Toe Pose)

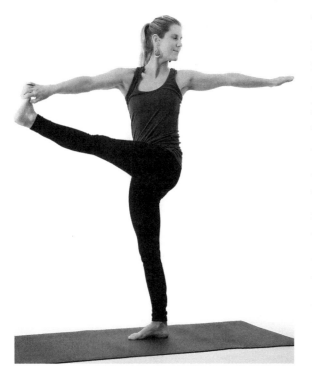

Verbally cue and demonstrate either lifting the right knee up from Tadasana or transitioning from Virabhadrasana III to lifting the torso and drawing the lifted leg through, then drawing the left hand across to clasp either the knee, along the leg, or eventually the foot. Many students will compromise the stable grounding of their standing leg by bending it or will compromise the elongation of their spine by folding to clasp farther toward the lifted foot. Encourage students to be more interested in keeping the standing leg straight and strongly engaged and their spine tall rather than attempting to clasp out so far. Emphasize pada bandha to help stabilize the standing ankle.

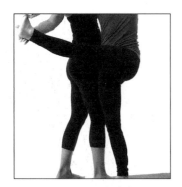

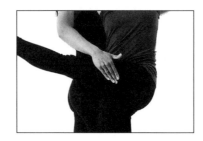

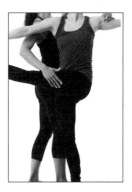

Stand on the student's standing-leg side facing opposite the direction the student is facing with Hip Stance to stabilize balance and upright posture.

Use Open Palm on the lifted leg to stabilize its positioning.

Use Open Palm on the shoulder of the side the student is twisting toward to assist rotation of the torso. This same hand can be used to help align the arm level with the floor and to encourage the shoulder blades down the back.

Modification

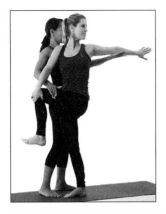

If the student is unable to keep the standing leg straight and the torso fully upright while clasping the lifted foot, encourage clasping a strap around the lifted foot or along that leg, or suggest bending and clasping the knee.

Explore Further

Teaching Yoga: pages 184-85
Yoga Sequencing: pages 406-7
Teaching Yoga Resource Center:
    www.markstephensyoga.com/resources

Garudasana Prep (Eagle Prep Pose)

Start in Tadasana and instruct students to slightly bend their knees, then either lift and cross their right ankle to their left knee (strongly flexing the ankle to stabilize the right knee). Then extend the arms wide apart to expand across the chest and upper back before crossing the left elbow over the right elbow and drawing the palms together (if it's not accessible, clasp that thumb or use the right hand to bring the left arm directly across the chest).

Encourage students to bend their knees more deeply both to stabilize their balance and to deepen the stretch of the external rotators of the hips while lifting the elbows level with the shoulders and squeezing the elbows together to deepen the stretch between their shoulder blades, keeping the spine tall, the heart center spacious, and the hands pressing away from the face.

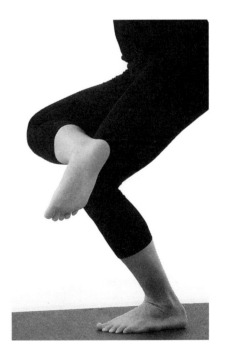

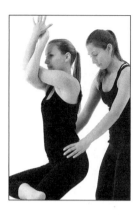

Use Hip Handles with Clasping Rotation to cue pelvic neutrality.

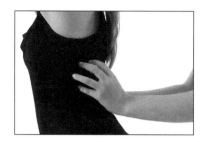

Use Finger Spreads to cue greater lengthening up through the spine.

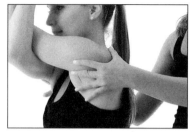

Use Opposite Rotation to cue lifting the arms (elbows up to level with the shoulders) and the shoulder blades down against the back ribs.

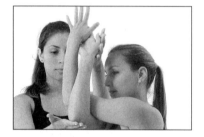

Use Open Palms and Light Touch to further cue the elbows up in line with the shoulders and the hands away from the face.

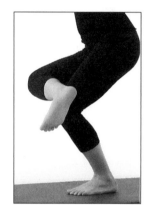

Introduce this asana with the ankle at the knee in strong dorsiflexion to help protect the knee. Students can maintain this position if unable to fully cross the knees in full Garudasana.

Explore Further

Teaching Yoga: page 183

Yoga Sequencing: page 386

Teaching Yoga Resource Center:
www.markstephensyoga.com/resources

Garudasana (Eagle Pose)

Teach in stages: bend the knees slightly, reaching the arms out with elbows bent down and the chest expanding; lift and cross the right ankle on the left knee, flexing the foot to stabilize the right knee, or, if possible, draw the knee all the way across the left knee and hook the right foot behind the left ankle or calf; reach out through the arms, then cross the left elbow over the right, drawing the forearms up and palms together (or try to clasp the right thumb), keeping the breath and the gaze steady. Try to lift the elbows level with the shoulders while drawing the shoulder blades down the back and pressing the hands away from the face; deepen the stretch between the shoulder blades by pressing the elbows and palms more firmly together. Try to bend the knees more deeply while lifting the spine and chest. If necessary, use a wall for added support.

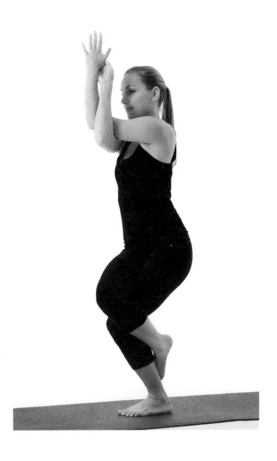

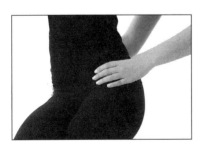

Use Hip Handles to assist balance and cue pelvic neutrality in relation to the lumbar spine.

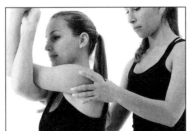

Use Opposite Rotation to cue the shoulder blades down the back and lifting of the arms (if possible extending your fingers just under the student's upper arms).

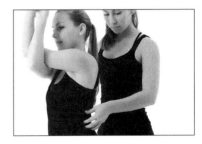

Use Finger Spreads to cue elongation of the spine by lifting the ribs up away from the pelvis.

Modification

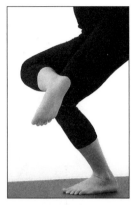

If unable to fully cross the knees, keep the ankle crossed just to the knee while keeping that foot strongly flexed to protect that knee.

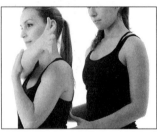

If unable to fully cross the elbows, use the lower arm to help draw the upper arm across the chest.

Explore Further

Teaching Yoga: page 183

Yoga Sequencing: page 386

Teaching Yoga Resource Center:
www.markstephensyoga.com/resources

Ardha Baddha Padmottanasana
(Half Bound Lotus Intense Stretch Pose)

From Tadasana, lift the right knee, cradle the lower leg, and draw the right heel toward the left hip (the anterior superior iliac spine or ASIS), then release through the inner right groin to allow the right knee to release down into a half-lotus position. Draw the right hand around behind the back to clasp the lotus foot. Reach the left arm straight up, then slowly fold forward and down as for Uttanasana. Inhaling, lift as for Ardha Uttanasana, then exhaling, fold back down and hold for five to eight breaths. To come up, inhaling, lift to the Ardha positioning, stay to exhale and feel the belly draw to the spine, then use that support inhaling back up to standing. Keep the standing leg strong and steady, bending the knee to take it easier on the hamstrings and lower back. Be very sensitive to the lotus knee, especially while folding forward, as this increases the potential twisting of the knee.

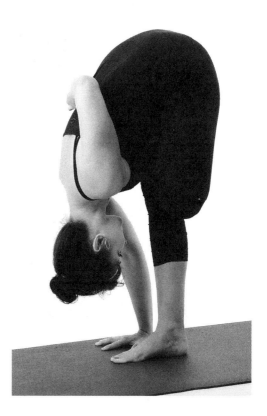

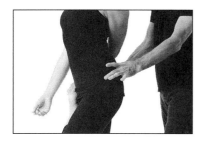

Use Hip Handles to cue balance and pelvic neutrality while being sensitive to the added pressure this may bring to the lotus knee.

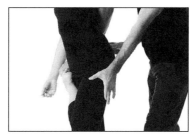

Apply Clasping Rotation to cue external rotation of the lotus thigh while being sensitive to added pressure in the knee.

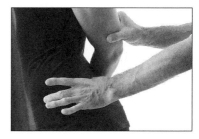

Apply Clasping Rotation to cue internal rotation of the arm clasping the lotus foot.

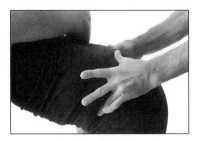 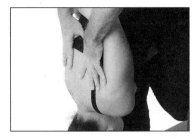 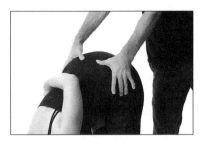

Use Clasping Rotation to cue anterior rotation of the pelvis as the initial and primary source of the forward fold while verbally cueing sensitivity to the lower back and hamstrings.

Use Opposite Rotation at the shoulder blades to cue the shoulder blades down the back and the sternum away from the belly.

Use Clasping Rotation to assist and cue posterior rotation of the pelvis as the action initiating movement back up to standing.

Modification

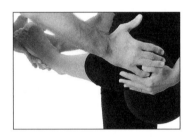

If unable to comfortably position the leg in the half-lotus position, explore cradling the lower leg while keeping the foot strongly flexed to protect the knee.

Explore Further

Teaching Yoga: page 185

Yoga Sequencing: pages 365-66

Teaching Yoga Resource Center:
www.markstephensyoga.com/resources

Chapter 5

Abdominal Core Integration

AN AWAKENED AND INTEGRATED ABDOMINAL CORE is a key source of support for the lumbar spine, allows us to more easily find levity in arm balances and floating movements, and opens us to moving more gracefully amid the challenges and opportunities in life. In popular fitness culture, the ideal core is often symbolized by "six-pack abs," referring to the rectus abdominis muscles that are the most superficial of the abdominal core muscles. When so overdeveloped and tight, rectus abdominis is a source of compressed tension as well as spinal and breathing problems, compromising the grace and ease, poise and elegance, comfort and stability that come from a refined core. As yoga teacher Ana Forrest has long emphasized, we want to relieve emotional and physical constipation and restriction, release deep guttural anxiety, not seal it in. Reminding students that yoga is largely about creating space, we want to guide students into cultivating a strong yet supple core, learning along the way to radiate outward while drawing awareness deep into the core of the body. As the core is strengthened, opened, and refined, it becomes a source of balance, stability, ease, and levity.

Taking an expanded view of the core, offer students a visual that extends from the medial arches of the feet awakened through pada bandha, up the inseams of the legs to the floor of the pelvis, up through the spine, and out through the crown of the head. Then, throughout the asana practice, encourage students to draw energetically in toward the medial line while radiating out from it to create space. Refer to pada bandha and mula bandha as key energetic actions for awakening this energetic awareness. This in itself will help to strengthen and refine the muscles that are at the heart of core refinement and make the more specific core awakening practices more accessible and sustainable.

Core awakening practices generally warm the body while bringing more targeted warming to the spine, pelvis, belly, and back, giving balanced awakening to all major abdominal core muscles: rectus abdominis, internal and external obliques, transversus abdominis, and iliopsoas. Core awakening is ideally explored just before arm balances, creating an awakened source of levity in asanas such as Bakasana (Crane Pose) and stability in poses such as Adho Mukha Vrksasana (Handstand). Focus more on awakening the rectus abdominis and iliopsoas in preparation for Bakasana, Urdhva Kukkutasana (Upward Rooster Pose), Galavasana (Flying Crow Pose), and other arm balances in which the pelvis is being lifted higher than the shoulders, and more on awakening the transversus abdominis and oblique muscles in preparation for Parsva Bakasana (Side Crane Pose), Astavakrasana (Eight-Angle Pose), and other arms balances in which the torso is being twisted. After working intensively with the iliopsoas in asanas such as Paripurna Navasana (Full Boat Pose), stretch it out before exploring Adho Mukha Vrksasana in order to minimize anterior rotation of the pelvis.

It can feel really good to stretch the belly immediately after a long and sustained abdominal core practice. Do this initially with simple spine and belly neutralizing twists, and never sequence deep back bends immediately following deep abdominal core strengthening practices—even though it may feel good at first. If core work is done prior to back bends, first neutralize the core through a sequence of simple twists, then after back bends, do core integration work to bring renewed support to the lumbar spine.

Mula Bandha and Uddiyana Bandha

Earlier we looked at the cultivation of pada bandha, the energetic awakening of the feet through the stirrup-like effect of contracting the tibialis posterior and peroneus longus muscles on the lower leg. The fascial attachments of these two muscles interweave with those of the hip adductors, which have origins in and around the ischial tuberosities (the sitting bones). The sitting bones are the lateral aspects of the pelvic floor, with the pubic symphysis at the front and the coccyx at the back. The front half of this diamond is the urogenital triangle, a landmark for the urogenital diaphragm, a hammock-like layer that is created by three sets of muscles: transverse perineal (connecting the two sitting bones), bulbospongiosus (surrounding the vagina or bulb of the penis), and ischiocavernosus (connecting the ischium to the clitoris or covering the penile crura) (Aldous 2004, 41). Contracting this set of muscles awakens the levator ani muscle, another hammock-like layer composed of the coccygeus, iliococcygeus, and the pubococcygeus muscles. When these muscles contract, they pull the entire pelvic floor up and naturally stimulate the awakening of core abdominal muscles with attachments at the pubis (in particular the transversus abdominis and rectus abdominis). This is the muscular action of mula bandha, which creates a feeling of grounded levity in the asana practice, supports the pelvic organs, creates an upward movement of energy, and stimulates uddiyana bandha. With practice, mula bandha can be accessed directly—independently of pada bandha—and steadily yet lightly maintained throughout asana practice without ever bearing down.

Uddiyana bandha is among the most misunderstood aspects of practice, owing in part to very different definitions and instructions from different traditions and teachers. In its full form, uddiyana bandha involves pulling the entire abdominal region strongly back toward the spine and then up toward the breastbone when completely empty of breath. Its engagement is part of specific pranayama and kriya practices, not asana practice, yet many teachers unfortunately instruct students to engage it while doing asanas. In asana practice we want the breath to flow smoothly, continuously, and fully, which requires the full, natural functioning of the diaphragm. However, uddiyana bandha prevents the diaphragm from expanding naturally, thus severely restricting the inhalation of breath.

The confusion about uddiyana bandha arises from a very different breath-related muscular action in the lower abdomen that we do want to cultivate in asana practice. With each and every complete exhale, the major abdominal muscles naturally contract (primarily the transversus abdominis but also the obliques and the rectus abdominis). When this occurs along with mula bandha, the very light, subtle engagement of these abdominal muscles can accentuate, deepen, and give more stability and ease to the body in many (but not all) asanas and asana transitions. Indeed, in some asanas we want the belly to be quite relaxed in order for the spine, pelvis, and breath to move appropriately for those asanas. We can refer to this as "uddiyana bandha light" to distinguish it from the full form of uddiyana bandha done in parts of pranayama practice.

Mula bandha and uddiyana bandha are tools that can be variously engaged to support different energetic actions in the practice. In no situation do we want to grip the belly as in full uddiyana bandha, which restricts the breath in asana practice. Nor do we want to create tightness in the pelvic floor. Rather, mula bandha and uddiyana bandha are best cultivated as light and steady energetic lifting actions that draw energy up and into the core of the body while allowing that energy to radiate out and fuel the practice. The balance of the qualities comes with practice, and with time it is increasingly subtle yet pervasive in its effects.

Here we will focus on asanas and dynamic movements designed to strengthen muscles in the front and center body that give support and mobility to the lower torso in its relationship to the pelvis and spine. (Contraction back bends and a variety of dynamic movements in and out of asanas will strengthen the muscles giving essential support to the spine from the back of the body.) Deep and sustained core awakening practices are largely contraindicated for pregnant students and should be approached very gingerly by students with lower-back issues.

Jathara Parivartanasana (Revolving Twist Pose)

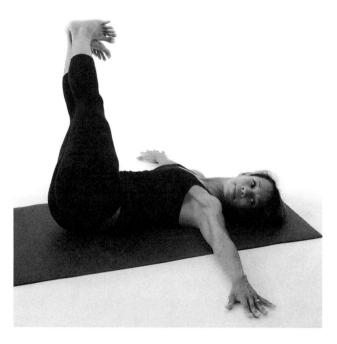

The basic form of this asana can be either a held twist (Supta Parivartanasana, Reclined Revolved Pose) or an abdominal core-strengthening movement. With the arms extended out like a cross and palms pressing down, cue students to alternately move the legs (or bent knees) back and forth to the left and right while gazing in the direction opposite the legs, keeping the knees or legs from touching the floor. Inhaling, extend the legs over; exhaling, draw them back up to center. Press the shoulders and palms firmly down while moving the legs, going only so far in the rotation as feels comfortable on the lower back.

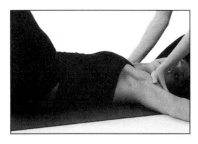

Use Light Touch on the shoulders and arms to cue their active grounding.

Modification

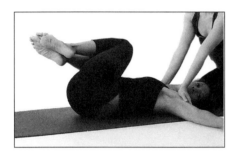

If the student strains with this movement, cue to keep the knees bent and to limit how far the knees are revolved from side to side.

Explore Further

Teaching Yoga: page 186

Yoga Sequencing: page 390

Teaching Yoga Resource Center:
www.markstephensyoga.com/resources

Tolasana (Scales Pose)

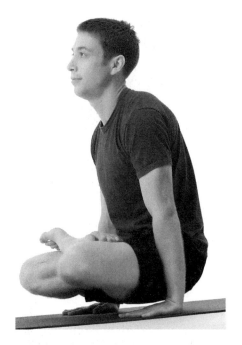

From Padmasana (Lotus Pose) or Sukhasana (Simple Pose, the simple cross-legged sitting position), place the hands on the floor by the hips. Gazing up, with the exhalation, press the hands down to lift off the floor (or try!) and hold while breathing. Focus on lifting straight up off the floor. To add intensity, do kapalabhati pranayama.

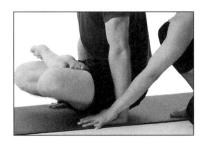

Use Light Touch to cue active grounding of the index fingers.

Modification

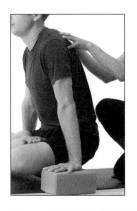

Place blocks under the hands to ease lifting off the floor, especially for students who are unable to place their palms firmly into the floor with bent elbows while sitting tall through the spine and torso.

Explore Further

Teaching Yoga: page 188

Yoga Sequencing: page 433

Teaching Yoga Resource Center:
   www.markstephensyoga.com/resources

Lolasana (Dangling Earring Pose)

From Vajrasana (Thunderbolt Pose), instruct students to cross their ankles and place their hands on the floor by their thighs. Gazing up, with the exhalation, press the hands down while arching the spine up, drawing the knees toward the chest and eventually the heels toward the tailbone. With practice, cue moving fluidly from Dandasana (Staff Pose) to Tolasana to Lolasana to Chaturanga Dandasana (Four-Limbed Staff Pose). More advanced students can transition from Lolasana to Adho Mukha Vrksasana.

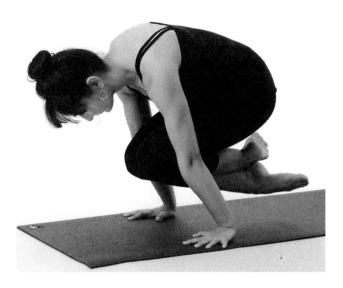

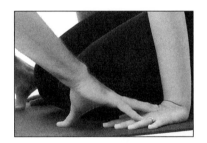

Use Light Touch to cue active grounding of the index fingers.

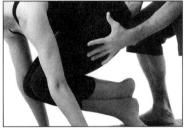

To assist a student in lifting up, keep your knees bent and your elbows on your knees while clasping the hips to help the student lift and center the weight over the hands.

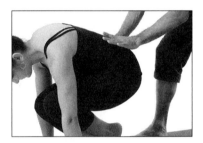

Use Light Touch to cue lifting the hips only as high as the shoulders.

Explore Further

Teaching Yoga: page 189

Yoga Sequencing: page 396

Teaching Yoga Resource Center:
   www.markstephensyoga.com/resources

Paripurna Navasana (Full Boat Pose)

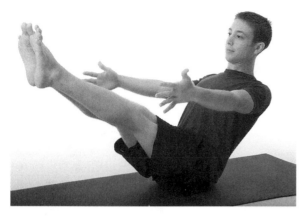

From Dandasana, instruct students to slide one heel back toward the hip on the same side, clasping that knee to leverage the anterior rotation of the pelvis while sitting taller, then draw in the other heel, clasping behind both knees while leaning slightly back. Maintaining the weight on the front of the sitting bones, slowly lift the feet off the floor, eventually straightening the legs and bringing the toes level with the eyes without slumping in the spine. Gradually hold less strongly with the hands, eventually extending the arms forward. Emphasize pelvic neutrality in relation to the spine and a spacious heart center. If able to straighten the legs, press out through the balls of the feet, spreading the toes and internally spiraling the thighs. For Ardha Navasana (Half Boat Pose), release the lower back to the floor, palms to the heart in anjali mudra, knees either in (easier) or straight legs about one foot off the floor. Add kapalabhati pranayama to intensify.

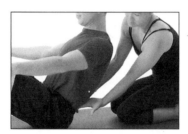

Use Light Touch to the lower back to cue the forward rotation of the pelvis into neutrality.

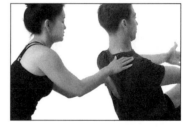

Use Light Touch with one hand on top of a shoulder and the other between the shoulder blades to cue lifting the spine up into the heart.

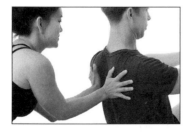

Use Finger Draws to cue the shoulder blades down against the back ribs while verbally cueing lifting the sternum.

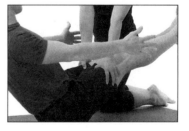

Use Clasping Rotation at the thighs to cue their internal rotation.

Explore Further

Teaching Yoga: page 188

Yoga Sequencing: page 401

Teaching Yoga Resource Center:
    www.markstephensyoga.com/resources

Dwi Chakra Vahanasana (Yogic Bicycles)

From Apanasana (Wind-Relieving Pose), interlace the fingers and cup the head in the hands. With the exhalation, curl the torso up, drawing the elbows toward the knees while extending the right leg straight out about one foot off the floor and extending the right arm out over the right leg. Complete the exhalation while drawing the right

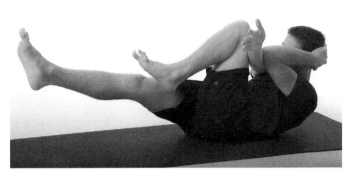

arm across the left knee and drawing the elbows together. Inhaling, release down, drawing the knees toward the chest and head and the elbows to the floor. Repeat on the other side, continuing for one to three minutes.

Emphasize moving slowly and working as low, deep, and broadly through the belly as possible. Encourage students to be more interested in moving slowly yet steadily rather than seeing how many they can do with a timed sequence. Move with the breath.

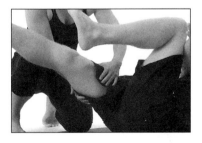

Use Light Touch on the thigh of the extended leg to cue its internal rotation.

Explore Further

Teaching Yoga: page 187

Yoga Sequencing: page 456

Teaching Yoga Resource Center:
    www.markstephensyoga.com/resources

Palavi Abhinatasana (Pelvic Tilts)

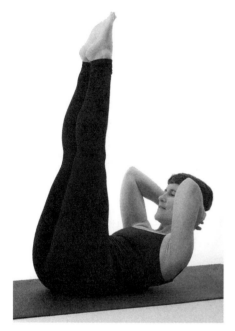

From Apanasana, extend the legs straight up, interlace the fingers, and cup the head in the hands. Keeping the legs vertical, on the exhalation, draw the elbows toward the knees without changing the position of the legs. Keeping the upper back and shoulders lifted, with each exhale, very slowly and smoothly curl the tailbone up, releasing it down as the breath flows out. Repeat five to twenty-five times. Students tend to focus on jerking the tailbone up. Encourage them to be more interested in slow and smooth movement than in maximizing the pelvic tilt. Emphasize keeping the legs vertical rather than drawing them toward the elbows.

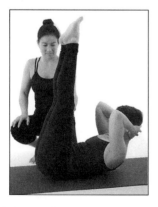

Use Light Touch to cue vertical positioning of the legs.

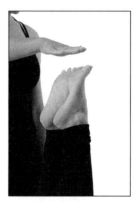

Place a palm above the student's toes to cue the direction of lift.

Explore Further

Teaching Yoga: page 187

Yoga Sequencing: pages 61-62

Teaching Yoga Resource Center:
   www.markstephensyoga.com/resources

Chapter 6

Arm Support and Balance

BALANCING THE ENTIRE BODY ON THE HANDS requires absolute focus, bringing students deeper into the meditative quality of *dharana* in their asana practice. Arm balances also bring students closer to a deeply held and perfectly rational fear of falling, a fear that is inextricably interwoven with the ego and the desire at least to appear in control. This makes arm balances the perfect asana family for cultivating self-confidence and humility. Because most students will find at least some arm balances very challenging, these asanas are also a wonderful place to explore the practice with a sense of humor and playfulness.

As with any asana, patience and practice make them more accessible and sustainable, while impatience almost invariably leads to frustration or injury. The wrists are at greatest risk in all arm-support asanas. Students with acute wrist issues, including carpal tunnel syndrome, should not do full arm balances, while students with even mildly strained wrists are advised to minimize pressure on the wrists and use a wedged hand prop until they are free of pain. Whether interspersing arm support asanas throughout practice or teaching them as a cluster of asanas, it is important to offer students the wrist therapy exercises described in the Healthy Wrist Sequence in *Yoga Sequencing*. Students should have sufficient wrist extension to place their palms flat on the floor and move their forearms perpendicular to the floor without strain or pain before attempting any arm balances.

Students with weak, unstable, or impinged shoulders are advised to do the Healthy Shoulder Sequence in *Yoga Sequencing* until developing sufficient stability and flexibility in the shoulder girdle to hold Adho Mukha Svanasana

(Downward-Facing Dog Pose) for two minutes free of pain before attempting more shoulder-intense arm balances. Limited shoulder flexion is also the primary cause of a banana shape to the spine in Adho Mukha Svanasana and Pincha Mayurasana (Feathered Peacock Pose or Forearm Balance). Along with strength and stability in the wrists, arms, and shoulders, arm balances require and awaken the abdominal core muscles.

As discussed above, abdominal work prior to arm balances helps students create a feeling of lifting and radiating out from their core. Yet arm balances also require suppleness in the core, not gripping or bearing down. Finding this balance between active engagement and spreading through the core is one of the key elements to balancing the body on the hands. This is most evident in Adho Mukha Vrksasana (Handstand), where strong core muscles stabilize the center of the body but where tight core muscles, especially in the psoas and rectus abdominis muscles, limit full extension of the hips and spine in relation to the pelvis, exacerbating the forward rotation of the pelvis and the banana shape in a student's lower back.

Adho Mukha Svanasana (Downward-Facing Dog Pose)

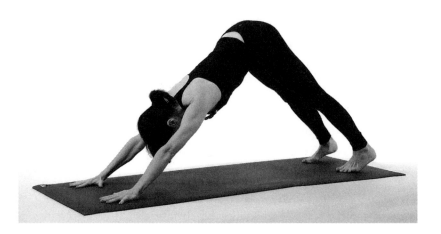

Adho Mukha Svanasana is the foundational asana for all other arm support asanas and is an excellent asana for learning and embodying the principle of roots and extension. Following the basic principles of asana practice, instruct Down Dog from the ground up and from what is at most risk of strain or injury: the wrists, shoulders, and hamstrings. We will look alternatively at the upper body (from the hands up) and the lower body (from the feet up).

Cue students to press firmly down into the entire span of their hands and the length of their fingers, paying close attention to rooting the knuckle of the index finger as a way of balancing pressure in the wrist joint. This rooting action should originate at the top of the arms. With it, ask students to feel the "rebounce" effect of this rooting action in the natural lengthening through their wrist, elbow, and shoulder joints. The fingers should be spread wide apart, the thumbs only about two-thirds of the way in order to protect the ligaments in the thenar space between the thumbs and index fingers. Generally, the middle fingers should be parallel and in line with the shoulders. Look to see if the student's arms are parallel; this will indicate if their hands are in line with their shoulders. The alignment of the wrists with the shoulders allows the proper external rotation of the shoulders, which activates and strengthens the teres minor and infraspinatus muscles (two of the four rotator cuff muscles), stabilizes the shoulder joint by drawing the scapulae firmly against the back ribs, creates more space across the upper back, and thereby allows the neck to relax more easily. If a student has difficulty straightening the arms, play with asking that person to turn the hands slightly out; if a student tends to hyperextend the elbows, have that person turn the palms slightly in.

Tight or weak shoulders create specific risks to the neck, back, elbows, wrists, and shoulders themselves in Down Dog. In either case, moderate effort in this asana develops both strength and flexibility, opening the shoulders to full flexion while developing deeper, more balanced strength. The shoulder blades should be rooted against the back ribs while spreading the shoulder blades out away from the spine. Note that externally rotating the shoulders tends to cause the inner palms to lift. This can be countered by internally rotating the forearms.

The roots-and-extension principle applies equally to the lower body. Rooting into the balls of the feet will contribute to lifting the inner arches, which is one effect of pada bandha (see chapter 4). This will help to stimulate the awakening of mula bandha (see chapter 5). The feet should be placed hip distance apart or wider, with the outer edges of the feet parallel. Firming the thighs and pressing the tops of the femur bones strongly back is a key action (along with rooted hands) in lengthening the spine in this asana. While firming the thighs, encourage students to slightly spiral the inner thighs back to soften pressure in the sacrum, all the while drawing the pubic bone back and up, the tailbone back and slightly down.

The first few times in this asana in any given practice, it can feel good and help the body in gently opening to "bicycle" the legs, twisting and sashaying alternately into each hip and stretching long through the sides of the body while exploring the hamstrings, lower back, shoulders, ankles, and feet.

Very flexible students tend to hyperextend their knees in Down Dog. Guide them to bend their knees slightly. Students with tight hips and hamstrings will find it difficult, painful, or impossible to straighten their legs. Encourage them to separate their feet wider apart (even as wide as their yoga mat) to ease the anterior rotation of the pelvis and the natural curvature of the lumbar spine. Let them know that it is okay to keep their knees bent while holding this asana, very gradually moving into deepening the flexibility of their hamstrings and other hip extensors.

With regular practice, the neck will become sufficiently strong and supple to support holding the head between the upper arms, with the ears in line with the arms. Until that strength is developed, encourage students to let their neck relax and their head hang. With each and every exhale, students will feel the light and natural engagement of their abdominal muscles. Encourage them to maintain that light and subtle engagement in their belly while inhaling, without gripping or bearing down in their belly. Keep bringing students' awareness back to the balanced ujjayi pranayama, to roots-and-extension, to a steady gaze, and to the cultivation of steadiness and ease.

In sum, in exploring Adho Mukha Svanasana, consider bringing the class to all fours to teach the fundamentals of the hands, arms, and pelvis, then lifting the hips up and back while moving toward straightening the legs. Healthy students with sufficient arm, shoulder, and core strength and stability can explore lifting the hips directly up and back into Adho Mukha Svanasana, either stepping over one foot at a time (relatively easier) or rolling over the toes on both feet simultaneously (more challenging). Many newer, very tight, or weak students are not prepared to safely practice full Adho Mukha Svanasana; they can stay on all fours to continue the preparatory work or explore the pose with their hands up a wall.

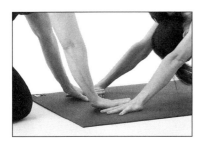

Use Light Touch to cue rooting the index fingers.

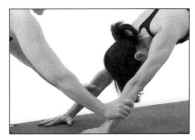

Use Clasping Rotation to cue internal rotation of the forearms.

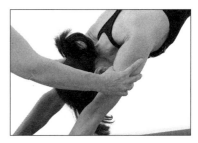

Use Clasping Rotation to cue external rotation of the arms.

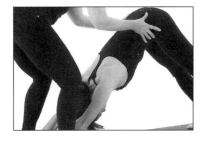

Use Hip Handles with Clasping Rotation to cue the pelvis into neutral alignment with the spine while pressing the pelvis away from the fingertips. (Do not press up if the student's knees are bent or if their heels are up high off the floor.)

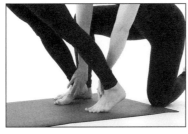

Use Finger Flicks to cue pada bandha and Light Touch to position the heels in straight alignment to the feet.

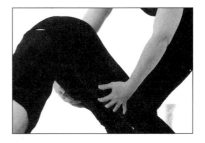

Use Light Touch to clarify or emphasize engaging the thighs and lifting the kneecaps.

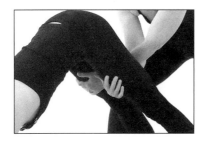

Use Crossed Wrists to cue internal rotation of the thighs and pressing of the thighs strongly back as the primary source of lengthening the spine.

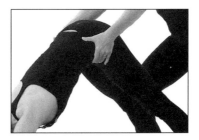

Use Hip Handles with Clasping Rotation to cue the pelvis into neutral alignment with the spine while pressing the pelvis away from the fingertips. (Do not press up if the student's knees are bent or if their heels are up high off the floor.)

Modification

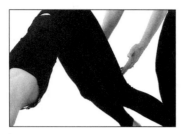

If the student rounds the lower back or the heels are up high off the floor, cue to bend the knees to take pressure away from the hamstrings and play with separating the feet as wide as the edges of the mat to ease rotation at the hips.

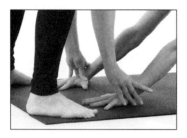

If the student hyperextends the elbows and can't help from doing so, cue to turn the hands slightly in. If the student is unable to fully extend the elbows, cue to turn the hands slightly out.

Explore Further

Teaching Yoga: page 164

Yoga Sequencing: page 360

Teaching Yoga Resource Center:
www.markstephensyoga.com/resources

Phalakasana (Plank Pose)

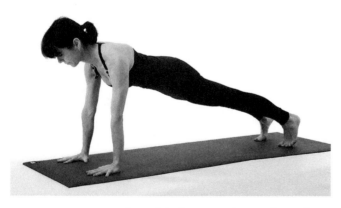

Phalakasana is a foundational asana that helps prepare students for all other arm-support asanas and is the basic preparatory position for the transition into Chaturanga Dandasana (Four-Limbed Staff Pose). It is contraindicated for students with significant wrist issues, and students with lower-back issues should keep their knees on the floor. Emphasize keeping the legs and core active to keep the pelvis from sagging, and cue firm pressure down through the palms and fingers while keeping the shoulder blades rooted down against the back ribs. Encourage students to look straight down or only slightly forward to help bring the sternum forward while keeping the neck comfortable.

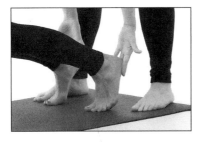

Place Light Hands on the heels to cue active rooting out through the heels.

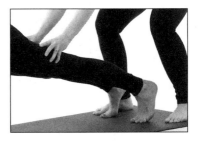

Use Clasping Rotation on the thighs to cue their slight internal rotation.

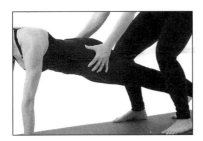

Use Hip Handles to cue the pelvis to a common plane with the shoulders and ankles and to help the student find pelvic neutrality.

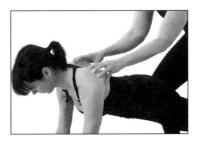

Cue the shoulder blades down the back with Finger Draws.

Modification

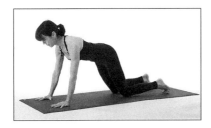

Place the knees on the floor until there is sufficient strength to hold the full asana for at least five breaths without straining.

Explore Further

Teaching Yoga: page 167-68

Yoga Sequencing: page 414

Teaching Yoga Resource Center:
www.markstephensyoga.com/resources

Chaturanga Dandasana (Four-Limbed Staff Pose)

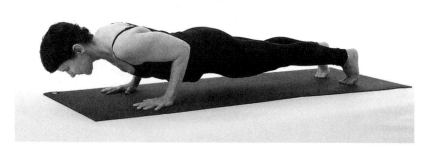

Prepare for Chaturanga in Phalakasana, teaching all of its elements. Cue students to keep their legs and core active and the sternum drawing forward as they slowly bend their elbows on an exhalation. Cue using the natural engagement of the abdominal muscles that happens with the exhalation to support the center of the body from sagging while lowering down. In lowering, cue students to align their elbows directly behind their shoulders without squeezing the elbows into their side ribs (although pressing into the side ribs can ease the transition for students still developing the strength to lower with stability and ease). Emphasize lowering only to where the shoulders are level with the elbows to reduce pressure in the front of the shoulders, all the while keeping the should blades rooted down against the back ribs, the chest spacious, and the sternum drawing forward. The gaze can be straight down to take it easier on the neck, or slightly forward to help cultivate a spacious heart center.

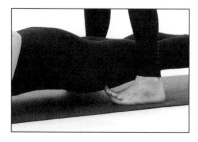

Place lifted toes under the student's thighs to cue activation of the legs while verbally cueing that activation.

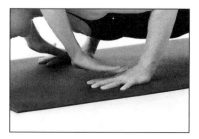

Press Light Hands onto the student's hands to emphasize their balanced rooting.

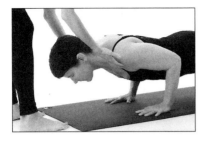

Place Light Hands under the student's shoulders at the level of the elbows as the student lowers while verbally cueing to lower to that position.

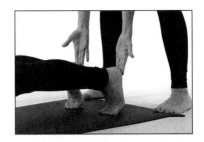

Press Light Hands against the student's heels while verbally cueing to press back through the heels.

Modification

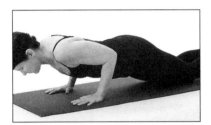

If the student lacks the strength to comfortably lower into Chaturanga, encourage the student to keep the knees on the floor while lowering down.

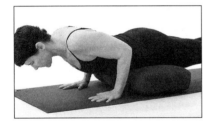

In introducing Chaturanga, place a high bolster under the student's torso and pelvis, then cue to press up off of it into Chaturanga before releasing slowly back onto the bolster, repeating several times while gradually cultivating the various energetic actions of full Chaturanga.

Explore Further

Teaching Yoga: page 167-68

Yoga Sequencing: page 377

Teaching Yoga Resource Center:
www.markstephensyoga.com/resources

Bakasana (Crane Pose)

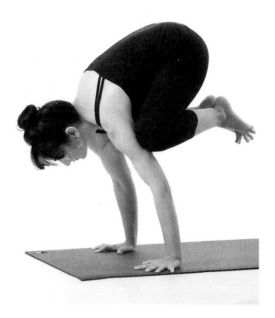

Bring students into a squat with the heels lifted and knees wide apart. Stretch the arms as far forward as possible, lengthening through the spine, shoulders, and arms, then slide the hands back under the shoulders while drawing the elbows outside the shins, thereby placing the knees as high onto the arms or shoulders as possible. Squeezing the knees into the arms or shoulders, press firmly into the hands and feet while lifting from the belly to elevate the hips as high as possible. Lean forward to bring the weight more into the hands, then begin to explore lifting the left and right feet alternately off the floor, eventually drawing both feet up together to the buttocks and straightening the arms. Place a stack of blankets under the face to reduce fear. Rooting firmly into the palms, with each exhalation renew the lifting of the belly toward the spine while drawing the pubic bone back and up. Keep the gaze steadily focused on a point directly beneath the head.

If stable, teach floating directly to Chaturanga Dandasana: creating a feeling of reaching the sternum toward the horizon, root more firmly through the hands, and with an exhalation, extend the feet directly back while bending the elbows to arrive in Chaturanga.

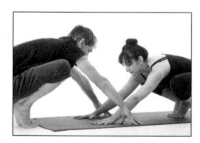

Verbally cue and demonstrate standing on the balls of the feet with the heels lifted and together, knees wide apart, and then stretching the arms forward and hands onto the floor, shoulder width apart.

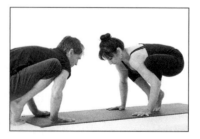

Verbally cue and demonstrate sliding the wrists beneath the shoulders and elbows outside the shins.

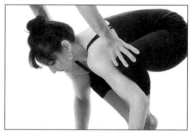

Use Light Hands to cue positioning the knees as high up the arms as possible.

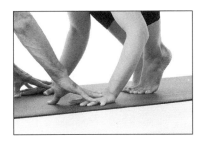

Use Light Hands to press the index fingers down.

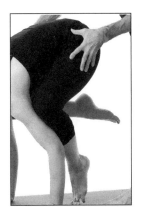

Verbally cue and demonstrate alternately lifting one foot then the other, either scissoring several times or eventually lifting both feet while rooting them firmly together. Use Hip Handles to assist lifting and balancing.

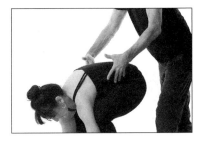

Use Light Hands to the belly to suggest activating the abdominal core as the primary source of lifting the hips.

Explore Further

Teaching Yoga: page 190

Yoga Sequencing: page 371

Teaching Yoga Resource Center:
    www.markstephensyoga.com/resources

Parsva Bakasana (Side Crane Pose)

Begin squatting as for Bakasana, come up high on the fingertips, straighten the legs halfway, twist from the torso, turn both knees to the left, and squat back down; then stretch the left arm up, press the knees farther back, and reach the left arm across the right knee (drawing the belly up and across the thigh), then place the left hand on the floor with both hands placed as though for Chaturanga Dandasana.

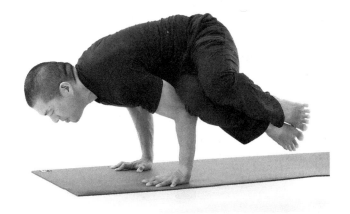

Rooting through the hands while lifting the sternum, begin tipping lightly forward on the tiptoes to bring the weight fully onto the hands, bending the elbows while reaching the sternum forward and keeping the ankles together as they lift off the floor. Keep rooting through the palms, keeping the elbows in line with the shoulders, knees even, breath and gaze steady. When stable, transition into Dwi Pada or Eka Pada Koundinyasana (Two-Leg or One-Leg Sage Koundinya's Pose). Each stage of this step-by-step approach offers something for everyone: a hip-opening squat, a twisting hip-opening squat, or a twisting arm balance.

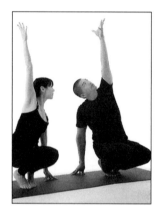

Verbally cue and demonstrate standing on the balls of the feet with the heels lifted and together, fingertips pressing into the floor under the shoulders, then straightening the legs halfway, twisting through the torso to point the knees ninety degrees to the right and then stretching the right arm up toward the sky.

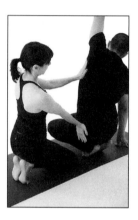

In Knees Down Stance behind the student, use Open Palms on the back ribs and side ribs to encourage lengthening up through the spine and the extended arm on an inhalation, then twisting to draw the right arm across the left knee on the exhalation, placing the palms on the floor with the fingers pointed forward.

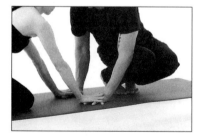

Verbally cue and demonstrate placing the left hand on the floor with the hands under the shoulders. Use Light Hands to cue pressing firmly down through the hands and fingers.

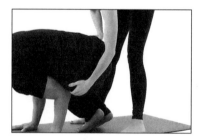

Verbally cue and demonstrate the option of placing the left hip on the left elbow as a prop; with practice, explore keeping the hip off the elbow.

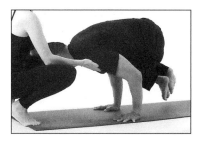

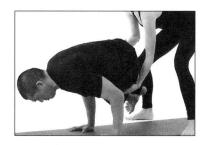

Verbally cue and demonstrate leaning forward into the hands while tipping off the tiptoes and bending the elbows to explore coming to balance on the hands. Use Open Palms to cue the shoulders level with elbows and the elbows from splaying out.

Use Horse Stance and Hip Handles while standing behind the student to assist with levity and balance.

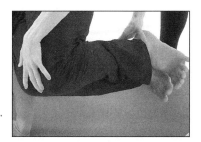

Use Light Hands to cue keeping the knees and ankles pressing together.

Explore Further

Teaching Yoga: page 191

Yoga Sequencing: page 411

Teaching Yoga Resource Center:
www.markstephensyoga.com/resources

Bhujapidasana (Shoulder-Squeezing Pose)

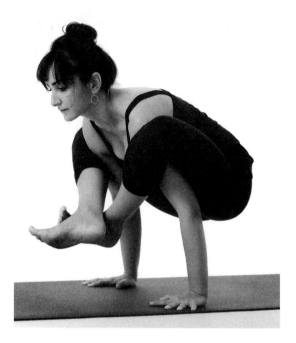

From Adho Mukha Svanasana, leap-frog the feet around the hands; slide the hands as far back as possible while keeping the wrists and palms rooted, positioning the knees against the shoulders. Squeezing the knees firmly into the upper arms or shoulders, release the hips slightly toward the floor to lift the feet off the floor more easily, then try to cross the ankles. If the knees are positioned at the shoulders, try to draw the heels to the buttocks and the top of the head to the floor, holding for five breaths or longer before transitioning back up.

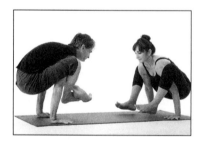

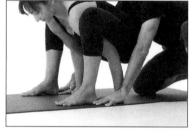

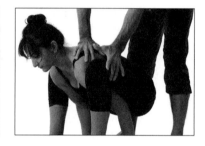

Verbally cue and demonstrate setting up either from Prasarita Padottanasana A (Spread-Leg Forward Fold Pose A), or from Adho Mukha Svanasana, leap-frogging the feet forward and outside the hands, then crawling the toes farther forward to position the knees as far up around the upper arms as possible.

Use light hands to cue pressing the hands and fingers firmly into the floor.

Use Open Palms to assist drawing the knees higher up the upper arms.

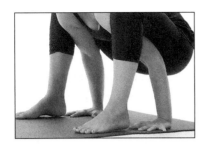

Verbally cue and demonstrate sitting back toward the elbows while lifting and crossing the ankles.

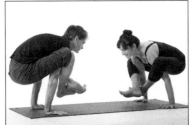

Verbally cue and demonstrate pressing more firmly down through the hands to press the arms straighter and lift the feet off the floor.

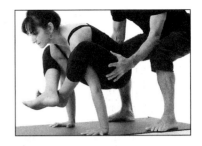

Use Hip Handles to assist lifting and balancing.

Modification

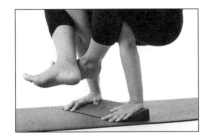

For students unable to place their hands fully on the floor, offer a wedge or blocks under their hands.

Explore Further

Teaching Yoga: page 192

Yoga Sequencing: page 375

Teaching Yoga Resource Center:
www.markstephensyoga.com/resources

Tittibhasana (Firefly Pose)

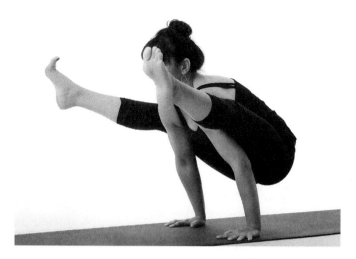

From Bhujapidasana, slowly extend the legs straight, spreading the toes and radiating out through the balls of the feet. Be very sensitive to the wrists, rooting more firmly through the knuckles of the index fingers. Intermediate students can try to transition to Bakasana, lifting the hips while drawing the heels out, back, and up.

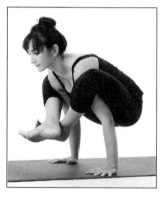

Verbally cue and demonstrate coming into Bhujapidasana.

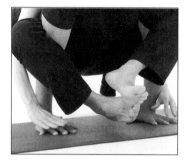

Verbally cue and demonstrate slowly extending the legs, pointing the feet, and spreading the toes. Use Light Hands to cue pressing the index fingers firmly down.

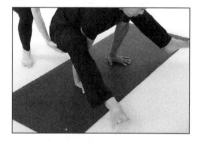

Use Hip Handles to assist the student in lifting the hips and straightening the arms while pressing the legs toward full extension.

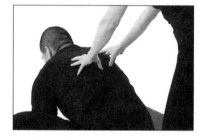

Use Finger Draws to cue the shoulder blades down the back while verbally cueing the student to lift the sternum.

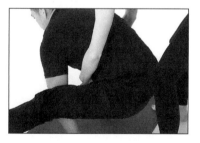

Use Light Hands to clarify and encourage active engagement of the belly in lifting the hips.

Modification

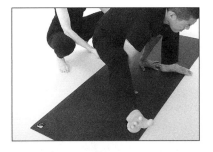

To prepare for Tittibhasana, start with Bhujapidasana and alternately extend and bend one knee and then the other.

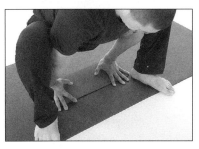

For students unable to place the palms firmly on the floor, offer a wedge under the hands. This also reduces pressure in the wrist joints.

Variation

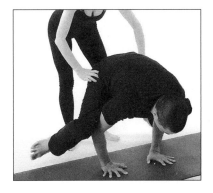

Use Hip Handles to assist the student in transitioning to Crane Pose.

Explore Further

Teaching Yoga: page 193

Yoga Sequencing: page 432

Teaching Yoga Resource Center:
  www.markstephensyoga.com/resources

Vasisthasana (Side Plank Pose or Side Arm Balance)

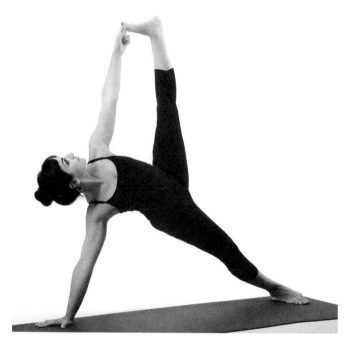

From Phalakasana, roll onto the outer edge of the left foot while drawing the right hand to the right hip. Placing the right ankle on top of the left ankle, flex both feet, and press the lower hip up. Rooting from the left shoulder through the left hand, explore either (a) sliding the right foot up the inner left thigh, as in Vrksasana (Tree Pose) or (b) clasping the left big toe and extending the left leg straight up. Keep the left hand and outer edge of the left foot firmly rooted. When lifting the right knee or leg, try to keep the right hip from moving either forward or back. Gaze up to the big toe, across toward the wall, or down to the floor.

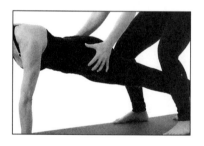

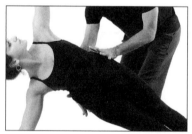

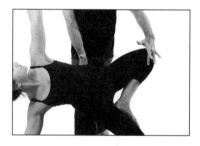

Verbally cue and demonstrate Phalakasana, then use Open Palms to cue the hips to be in line with the shoulders and ankles (neither sagging nor elevated).

Verbally cue and demonstrate shifting onto the outer edge of the right foot and stacking the ankles with both feet strongly flexed, again using Open Palms to cue the hips to be in line with the shoulders and ankles.

Standing behind the student with your leg braced lightly against their sacrum, verbally cue positioning the upper foot as though for Vrksasana without either sagging in the hips or allowing the upper hip to move back. Use an Open Palm on the bent knee to encourage the Vrksasana hip opening while using your leg to keep the student's upper hip from shifting back.

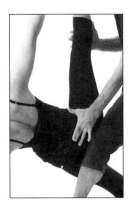 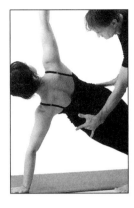 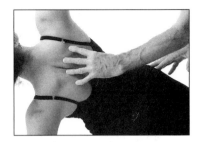

Verbally cue clasping the big toe of the upper foot in Vrksasana position and extending that leg, without either sagging in the hips or allowing the upper hip to move back. Use an Open Palm on the lifted leg to encourage the same hip opening while using your leg to keep the student's upper hip from shifting back.

If the student's lower hip is sagging, use a Light Hand to cue keeping it lifted.

Use Finger Draw to cue the shoulder blades down against the back ribs and expanding across the chest.

Modification

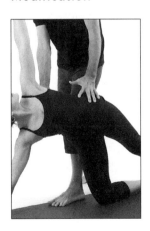

The basic modified position is to place the knee of the lower leg on the floor. The supporting hand can be placed farther ahead of the shoulder to reduce pressure in the wrist. Use Open Palms on the shoulders to cue the torso to face toward the wall (rather than collapsing toward the floor).

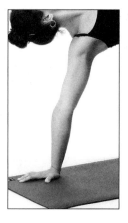

The supporting hand can be placed farther ahead of the shoulder to reduce pressure in the wrist. Placing the forearm on the floor eliminates any pressure on the wrist.

Explore Further

Teaching Yoga: page 196

Yoga Sequencing: page 448

Teaching Yoga Resource Center:
   www.markstephensyoga.com/resources

Eka Pada Koundinyasana A (One-Leg Sage Koundinya's Pose A)

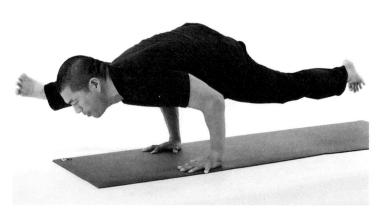

From the wrapped variation of Virabhadrasana II (Warrior II Pose) or from Ashta Chandrasana (Crescent Pose) prep, draw the right shoulder under the right knee, place the hands and arms as for Chataranga, and extend the right leg while tipping off the back foot to explore balancing on the hands. Gaze forward (or down to take it easier on the neck), keep the shoulders and ears level with the floor and, with an exhale, use light uddiyana bandha to gain levity in floating to Chataranga.

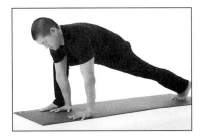 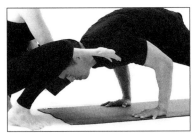 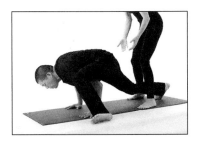

Begin in Ashta Chandrasana (Crescent Pose) or Utthita Parsvakonasana (Extended Side Angle Pose), then place the hands as for Chaturanga Dandasana.

Use Open Palms and Light Hands to cue the shoulders level with the elbows, as for Chaturanga.

Verbally cue and demonstrate using the back foot to tip the weight forward toward balance while extending the front leg forward and out to the side.

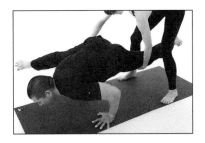 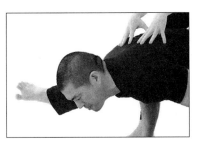 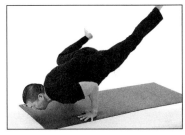

Straddling the student, use Open Palms on both legs to assist the student in extending back, hip height off the floor, and extending the front leg forward and out to the side.

Use Finger Draws to cue the shoulder blades down against the back ribs.

Verbally cue and demonstrate floating into Chaturanga on an exhalation.

Modification

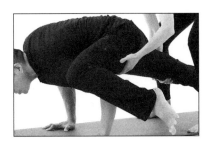

For students with tight hips and hamstrings, cue keeping the front knee bent while tipping forward off the back toes. Use the straddling technique to assist this movement.

Variation

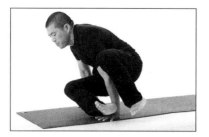

Transition directly into Astavakrasana (Eight-Angle Pose), then back into this asana before floating back into Chaturanga.

Explore Further

Teaching Yoga: page 195

Yoga Sequencing: page 381

Teaching Yoga Resource Center:
www.markstephensyoga.com/resources

Adho Mukha Vrksasana
(Downward-Facing Tree Pose or Handstand)

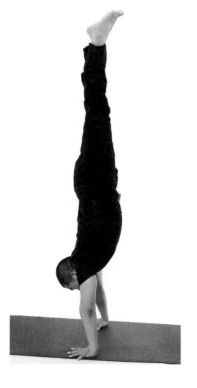

Introduce at a wall in three stages: (1) in an L shape (like Adho Mukha Svanasana) with the hands on the wall and the feet on the floor, alternately extending one leg up while maintaining all the qualities of Adho Mukha Svanasana in the upper body; (2) in an L shape with the hands on the floor under the shoulders and the feet on the wall where the hands just were, alternately extending one leg straight up; and (3) with the fingertips five inches from the wall. Extend one leg back and up, keeping it straight and strong; begin springing off the other foot while swinging the lifted leg up. The moment the springing leg is sprung, make it straight and strong, and draw it up next to the other leg overhead.

Pressing down firmly through the hands as in Adho Mukha Svanasana, first flex the feet and extend up through the legs and heels, then point and press out through the balls of the feet. While drawing longer through the core of the body, wrap the shoulder blades broadly as in Adho Mukha Svanasana, lightly engage the belly to support the stable connection of the torso and pelvis, keep the floating ribs in and away from the skin while pressing the tailbone and pubis up, activate mula bandha, spiral the femurs internally, and breathe while gazing down between the thumbs.

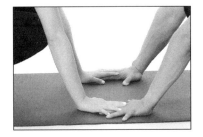

Use Light Touch to cue rooting the index fingers.

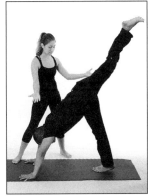

To assist in scissor-kicking up, take Horse Stance at a forty-five-degree angle to the student on the side of the lifted leg, with one arm extended across in line with the wrists (as a bar to prevent the student from going over) and the other prepared to assist the lifted leg in swinging up.

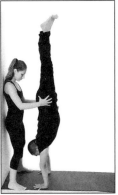

Once up, move behind the student and use firm Clasping Rotation at the hips to center the hips over the wrists and to assist in positioning the legs straight up.

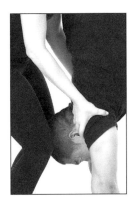

Once the student is in basic alignment (at a wall or in the middle of the room), give the finger, arm, and shoulder cues for Adho Mukha Svanasana.

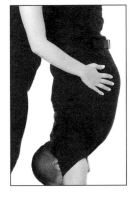

Use Light Hands on the lower front ribs to cue them in.

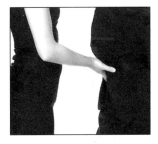

Use Light Hands on the sacrum to cue the pelvis into neutral position.

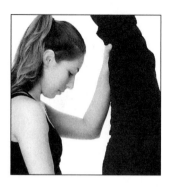

Place a hand between the student's knees for just the moment it takes to cue to make the two legs feel as though one.

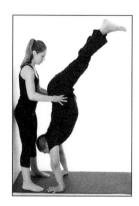

Use Clasping Rotation at the hips to ease the student down into an easy standing forward bend for a few breaths.

Modification

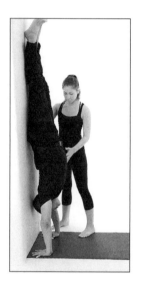

Use a wall for support. Also suggest staying with one of the preparatory positions.

Explore Further

Teaching Yoga: page 193

Yoga Sequencing: pages 361

Teaching Yoga Resource Center:
   www.markstephensyoga.com/resources

Shishulasana (Dolphin Pose)

Verbally cue and demonstrate, starting on all fours with the toes curled under, and then placing the forearms on the floor parallel to each other. If unable to keep the forearms parallel, either place blocks between the index fingers and a strap just above the elbows, or interlace the fingers and still consider using the strap. Cue rooting down through the hands and forearms while pressing the shoulders away from the wrists and lifting the hips up and back, pressing the legs gradually straight.

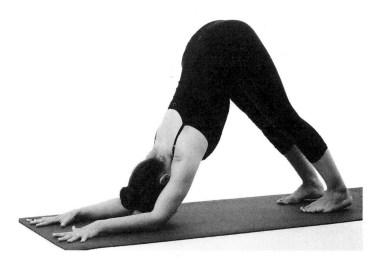

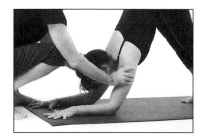

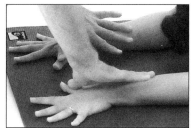

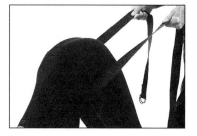

Use Clasping Rotation at the shoulders to cue their active external rotation, thereby stabilizing the shoulders and reducing pressure around the neck.

Use Light Hands on the hands and then the forearms to cue their internal rotation, thereby better rooting the hands and minimizing pressure in the wrists.

Place a strap across the upper thighs and pull it evenly up and back to cue bringing the weight more into the legs and thereby lengthening the spine.

Modification

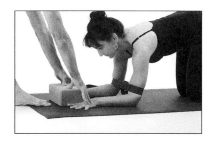

With the knees on the floor, explore the various arm positions and uses of props for the arms.

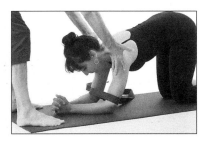

Cue the interlacing of the fingers to make the arm and shoulder positioning more accessible to students with tight shoulders.

Variation

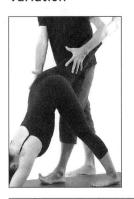

Cue extending one leg up and back, using Open Palms and Clasping Rotation to cue the hips level and the internal rotation and greater extension of the leg.

Explore Further

Teaching Yoga: page 194

Yoga Sequencing: page 427

Teaching Yoga Resource Center:
  www.markstephensyoga.com/resources

Pincha Mayurasana (Feathered Peacock Pose or Forearm Balance)

Use the same steps as described for introducing Adho Mukha Vrksasana, except the forearms are placed on the floor. If students' forearms splay, place a block between the index fingers and a strap just above the elbows. In stage 3, press the shoulders as far back from the wrists as possible. Maintain this positioning when scissor-kicking the legs up overhead. Once in Pincha Mayurasana, press firmly through the palms and elbows, drawing the shoulders away from the wrists while pressing the tailbone toward the feet and toward the ceiling. Internally rotate the femurs.

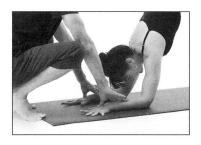

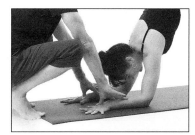

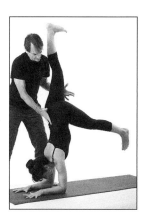

Prepare as for Shishulasana, using Light Hands to cue the firm rooting of the hands and fingers.

Verbally cue walking the feet closer to the elbows to position the hips over the shoulders, using Open Palms to emphasize rooting the inner hands and pressing the shoulders away from the wrists.

Verbally cue extending one leg up into scissor-kicking position, then further cue keeping that leg fully extended while swinging it up and simultaneously hopping off the other foot, making the hopping leg straight and strong as soon as it springs from the floor.

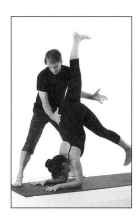

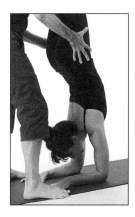

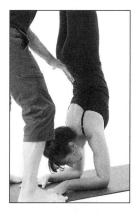

To assist in scissor-kicking up, take Horse Stance at a forty-five-degree angle to the student on the side of the lifted leg, with one arm extended across in line with the shoulders (as a bar to prevent the student from going over) and the other prepared to assist the lifted leg in swinging up.

Once up, move behind the student and use firm Clasping Rotation at the hips to center the hips over the shoulders and to assist in positioning the legs straight up.

Use Light Hands on the sacrum to cue the pelvis into neutral position.

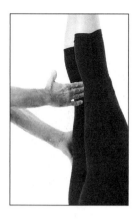

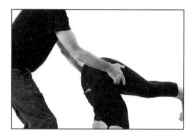

Place a hand between the student's knees for just the moment it takes to cue to make the two legs feel as though one.

Use Clasping Rotation at the hips to ease the student down.

Modification

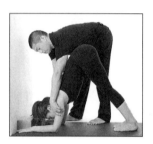

Practicing at a wall, place a block or blocks between the index fingers and/or a strap just above the elbows to keep the arms aligned, and verbally cue Shishulasana push-ups, using Open Palms to cue pressing the shoulders away from the wrists.

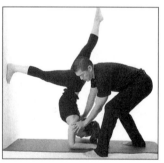

For an even more accessible position, place the forearms on the wall to develop the basic form and awareness of the asana. Use Open Palms to cue spreading the shoulder blades apart and down and away from the ears. For the next stage, practice in an L shape with the feet on the wall at hip height and the forearms on the floor, then playing with extending one leg straight up, then switching to the other leg.

Explore Further

Teaching Yoga: page 194

Yoga Sequencing: page 414

Teaching Yoga Resource Center:
www.markstephensyoga.com/resources

Astavakrasana (Eight-Angle Pose)

In Dandasana (Staff Pose), slide the right foot in, clasping the knee to leverage the anterior rotation of the pelvis and extension of the spine. Then: (1) clasp the right foot and move it around in a figure eight in front of the chest; (2) cradle the lower right leg between the elbows, flex the right foot, and rock the cradle; (3) draw the right knee over the right shoulder while reaching the right

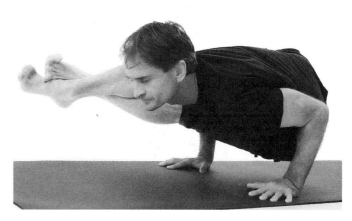

arm forward, placing the right palm next to the right hip, left palm by the left hip; (4) lift the left leg off the floor, then with an exhale, press through the hands to lift the hips off the floor; (5) cross the right ankle over the left ankle and extend the legs straight out to the left; (6) bend the elbows until the shoulders are level with them.

Keep rooting the palms, lifting the hips, pressing out through the balls of the feet, squeezing the knees toward each other, drawing the sternum forward, and gazing either down (easier on the neck) or to the horizon. Explore transitioning to Eka Pada Koundinyasana by (1) straightening the arms, (2) lifting the hips, (3) unhooking the feet, (4) threading the left foot and leg back between the arms, and (5) scissoring the legs apart. From there, float to Chaturanga.

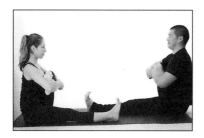

Verbally cue and demonstrate Dandasana, then draw one knee in as for Marichyasana A (Sage Marichi's Pose A), and then cradle that lower leg across the chest before bringing the knee over the shoulder and the hands back to the floor.

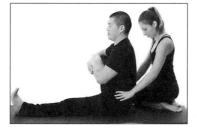

Use Hip Handles and Opposite Rotation at the hips to cue anterior rotation of the pelvis and use Light Hands up the back to suggest lengthening the spine.

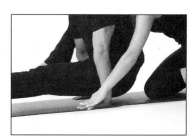

Verbally cue and demonstrate lifting the extended leg off the floor, then pressing the hands down to lift completely off the floor. Use Light Hands to press the index fingers down.

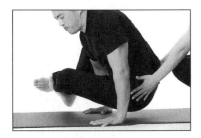

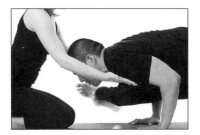

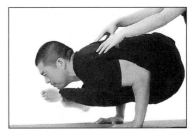

Verbally cue and demon-
strate crossing the ankle of the
extended leg over the other ankle,
then extending both legs straight
out to the side. Use Open Palms
at the hips to assist the student in
lifting up.

Verbally cue and demonstrate
slowly bending the elbows to
position the shoulders level with
the elbows. Use Open Palms to
cue the level positioning of the
shoulders.

Use Finger Draws to cue the
shoulder blades down the back.

Explore Further

Teaching Yoga: page 194

Yoga Sequencing: page 369

Teaching Yoga Resource Center:
    www.markstephensyoga.com/resources

Galavasana (Flying Crow Pose)

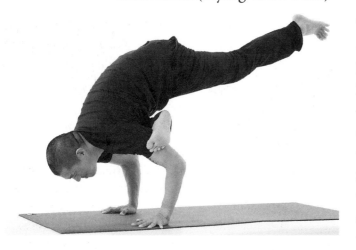

Teach in steps: (1) from Tadasana
(Mountain Pose), bend the knees, then
lift and cross the right ankle onto the
left knee, strongly flexing the right foot;
(2) draw the palms together at the heart
center; (3) bring the palms to the floor
under the shoulders, hooking the flexed
right foot around the left shoulder
while placing the left knee on the left
shoulder; (4) pressing the palms, lean
the weight forward; (5) extend the left
leg back and up. While rooting through the hands, draw the sternum forward and
press out through the extended left leg. Either float to Chaturanga or transition

into Sirsasana II (Headstand II) in preparation for transitioning directly to the other side of the asana.

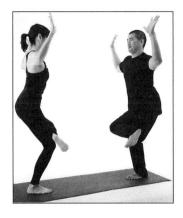

Starting in Tadasana, verbally cue and demonstrate bending one knee while placing the other ankle onto that knee and strongly flexing the foot in dorsiflexion to stabilized the lifted knee, and draw the palms together at the heart.

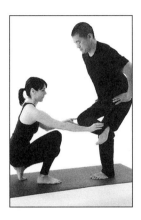

Use Light Hands to cue positioning of the ankle just above the knee (not up the thigh) and flexing of the ankle.

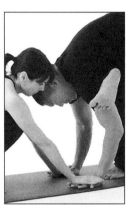

Verbally cue and demonstrate folding forward to place the hands on the floor, and use Light Hands to cue positioning the wrists under the shoulders and thereby bring the upper arms close to the crossed shin.

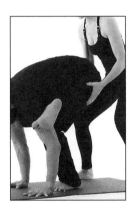

Verbally cue and demonstrate leaning into the hands while trying to press the arms straight, or assisting by standing to the side and using Hip Handles to help the student press the arms straighter.

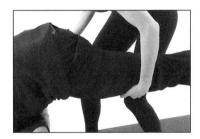

Verbally cue and demonstrate lifting the rooted foot off the floor and extending that leg back and up, or assist by standing to the side and helping to lift the hips.

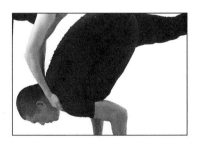

Once the student extends the leg back and up, use Open Palms at the shoulders to suggest pressing the arms straighter while balancing the weight of the body evenly over the hands.

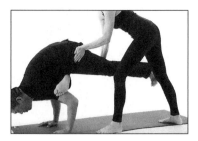

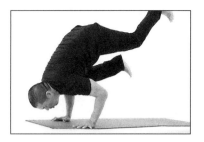

Use Open Palms on the outside of the extended hip and inner thigh of that leg to cue level hips and internal rotation and extension of the extended leg.

Verbally cue and demonstrate floating into Chaturanga on an exhalation.

Explore Further

Teaching Yoga: page 196

Yoga Sequencing: page 385

Teaching Yoga Resource Center:
www.markstephensyoga.com/resources

Urdhva Kukkutasana (Upward Rooster Pose)

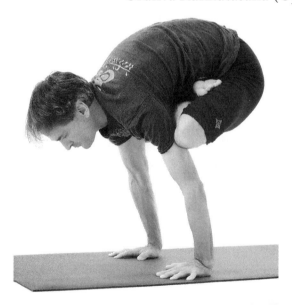

There are two basic ways in: (1) from Padmasana (Lotus Pose), press through the hands while standing on the knees, then, with an exhale, slide the knees up the arms; (2) from Sirsasana II, fold the legs into Padmasana position, lower the knees to the shoulders, and press the hands to straighten the arms.

Maintain pada bandha, mula bandha, and light uddiyana bandha. Gaze straight down. Transition to Chaturanga Dandasana or to Sirsasana II; from there, explore Parsva Kukkutasana (Side Rooster Pose) by twisting across as in Parsva Bakasana.

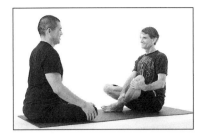

Verbally cue and demonstrate coming into Lotus Pose.

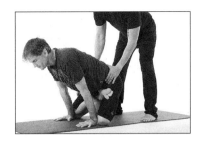

Use Hip Handles to assist the student in standing on the knees with the hands on the floor under the shoulders. Verbally cue pressing equally and firmly down through the hands while feeling the belly engage on the exhalations.

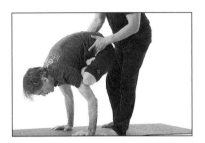

Use Hip Handles to assist the student in sliding the shins up the arms while exhaling, using the belly to create the elevation of the hips and positioning the shins as far toward the shoulders as possible. Use Hip Handles to assist the student in finding balance on the hands.

Variation

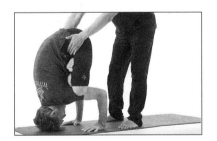

Use Hip Handles to ease the student's head to the floor for a Sirsasana II position, then cue pressing the knees overhead in preparation for Parsva Kukkutasana.

Explore Further

Teaching Yoga: page 197

Yoga Sequencing: page 437

Teaching Yoga Resource Center: www.markstephensyoga.com/resources

---

Uttana Prasithasana (Flying Lizard Pose)

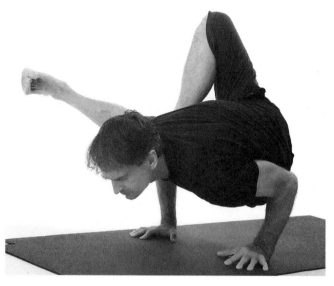

Come to step 2 of Galavasana prep, then: (1) use the left hand to stabilize the right ankle on the left knee; (2) stretch the right arm up to lengthen through the right side; (3) twist the torso and draw the right elbow to the left arch, pressing the palms together to leverage the twist; (4) draw the right shoulder to the arch and release the right hand to the floor outside the left ankle; (5) place the left hand on the floor, shoulder distance from the right hand; (6) lean the weight to the left while bending the elbows, extending the left leg to the left and off the floor, and reaching the chest forward. Instruct students to try to bring their shoulders level with each other. Energize out through the extended leg. Float to Chaturanga.

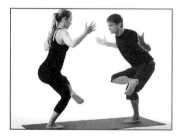

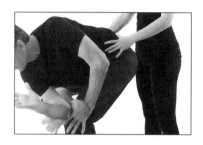

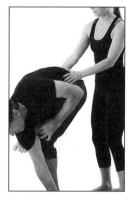

Verbally cue and demonstrate coming into the standing preparatory position for Galavasana, with the right ankle to the left knee.

Verbally cue and demonstrate placing the left hand on the right heel while stretching the right hand up overhead, then use Open Palms on the back-to-side ribs to encourage lengthening up through the spine and the extended arm on an inhalation, then twisting to draw the right elbow across the left knee on the exhalation for a prayer twist position.

Use Hip Handles to assist the student's balance, or if tall enough, straddle the student in a wide Mountain Stance and squeeze your knees onto the student's hips to free your hands to assist with Open Palms along the side ribs in deepening the twist until the student's right shoulder crosses the knee. This is the crux of the asana.

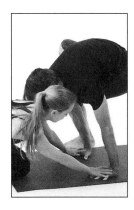

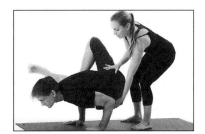

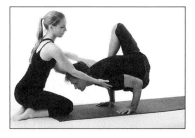

Verbally cue placing the right hand on the floor next to the right foot, then leaning to the left to place the left hand on the floor with the hands placed as for Adho Mukha Svanasana. Use Light Hands to cue equal pressure down through the hands and fingers.

Use Hip Handles to relieve weight from the student's arms and shoulders while verbally cueing to extend the left leg straight over to the right while bending the elbows as though for Chaturanga. The left leg should be resting on the upper right arm next to the right foot.

Use Light Hands or Open Palms to cue keeping the shoulders level and at elbow height.

Explore Further

Teaching Yoga: page 196

Yoga Sequencing: page 443

Teaching Yoga Resource Center:
   www.markstephensyoga.com/resources

Chapter 7

Back Bends

WITH DEEP STRETCHING ACROSS THE ENTIRE FRONT OF THE BODY, especially through the heart center, belly, and groin, back bends stimulate a passionate response among students. The passion tends to go toward either unbridled effort or fearful withdrawal, offering students another opportunity for cultivating equanimity amid these emotional poles.

The primary physical purpose of back bends is to open to the full movement of breath and energy in the front of the body, not to go into the most gloriously deep stretch of the front of the body. You can guide students into finding a sense of sustainable effort in playing the edge in their back-bend practice by emphasizing the heart opening qualities of this practice: feeling compassion toward oneself in feeling one's way toward the edge, opening to a sense of innate inner harmony as a source of aparigraha, sensing a healing presence within the breath that reinforces a sense of assessment rather than judgment, and recognizing the love in the heart as the glue that holds everything together in the unending process of change. Encourage back bends as a practice of equanimity, not attainment, and purification for the purpose of freedom, not perfection, focusing on opening the heart.

Asanas in the back-bend family can be usefully categorized into contraction, traction, and leverage back bends, each of which has important distinctions and actions:

- **contraction back bends:** Muscles along the back of the body concentrically contract to overcome gravity; for example, lifting up into Salabhasana A (Locust Pose A).

- **traction back bends:** Muscles in the front of the body eccentrically contract to overcome gravity; for example, lowering back into Ustrasana (Camel Pose).
- **leveraged back bends:** The arms and/or legs press against a stable object (the floor, a wall, or another part of the body) to stretch the front of the body; for example, Dhanurasana (Bow Pose) or Urdhva Dhanurasana (Upward-Facing Bow Pose).

Within each of these categories of back bends, the humerus can either be in extension or flexion. It is in extension in asanas such as Salabhasana A, Ustrasana, or Setu Bandha Sarvangasana (Bridge Pose); it is in flexion in asanas such as Salabhasana C, Kapotasana (Pigeon Pose), or Viparita Dandasana (Inverted Staff Pose). These different arm positions require different areas of engagement and release through the shoulder girdle, as follows:

- **shoulder extension back bends:** Extension of the arms requires the scapulae to be stabilized by the rhomboids, lower trapezius muscles, and serratus anterior muscles while the pectoralis majors and minors must release.
- **shoulder flexion back bends:** Flexion requires the rhomboids, latissimi dorsi, pectoralis majors, and triceps to release.

Salabhasana A, B, C (Locust Pose A, B, C)

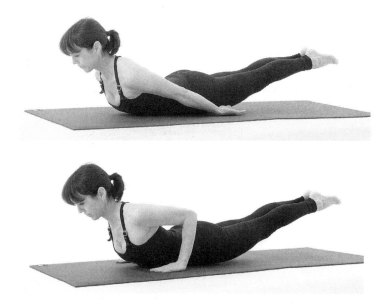

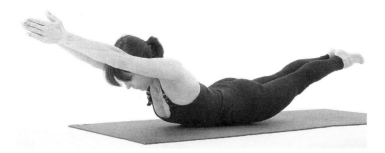

From Phalakasana (Plank Pose), sequentially bring the knees, chest, and chin to the floor (*ashtanga pranam,* or eight-point prostration) on the exhalation, then release completely onto the floor, grounding the hips and feet firmly into the floor, energetically extending back through the legs and feet, spiraling the inner thighs up, and pressing the tailbone toward the heels. While students maintain this active engagement of their legs, guide them into either A, B, or C as follows:

- A: Keep the backs of the hands pressing firmly into the floor to leverage the lifting of the chest and the feeling of bringing the thoracic spine forward and up into the heart center.

- B: Cue students to press into their hands—placed beneath their elbows— and lift their chest up while shrugging their shoulder blades down their back and looking slightly down to maintain ease in the neck.

- C: In variation C, emphasize keeping the shoulder blades rooted down against the back ribs while spiraling them broadly out as in Adho Mukha Svanasana (Downward-Facing Dog Pose).

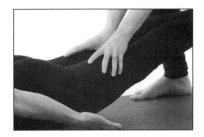

Use Light Hands to cue internal rotation of the thighs.

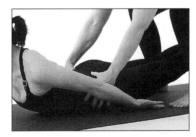

Use Hip Handles and Clasping Rotation to cue grounding and slight posterior rotation of the pelvis. Then cue the student to lift the legs off the floor (or not, if this creates tension in the lower back), and to fully extend the legs.

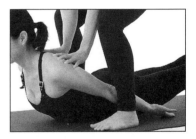

For Salabhasana A, use Finger Draws to cue the shoulder blades down the back while verbally cueing the action of bringing the mid-to-upper spine into the heart.

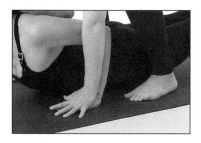

For Salabhasana B, place Light Hands on the student's hands to cue an outward spiraling without actually moving the hands, thereby helping to align the elbows behind the shoulders and to expand the chest.

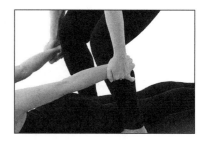

For Salabhasana C, start with the preparatory position with the fingers interlaced behind the back. If that's easily accessible and the student has a healthy lower back, take Horse Stance with your feet next to the hips and your elbows on your knees, then clasp the wrists to guide the hands to clasp around the top of your calves.

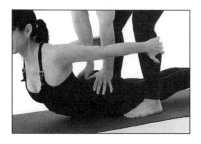

Still with Salabhasana C prep, now use Hip Handles and Clasping Rotation to cue grounding and slight posterior rotation of the pelvis while slowly pressing your legs straighter, thereby deepening the student's back bend. Firmly clasp the arms before gradually easing the student down, and only then ask the student to let go of your calves.

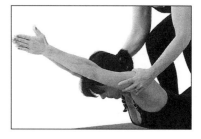

In the full expression of Salabhasana C, use Clasping Rotation of the student's upper arms to cue their external rotation.

Modification

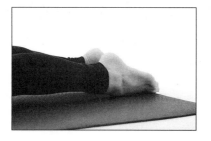

For Salabhasana A, B, or C, suggest keeping the feet actively rooted to the floor to take it easier on the lower back.

Explore Further

Teaching Yoga: pages 163-64
Yoga Sequencing: page 421
Teaching Yoga Resource Center: www.markstephensyoga.com/resources

Bhujangasana (Cobra Pose)

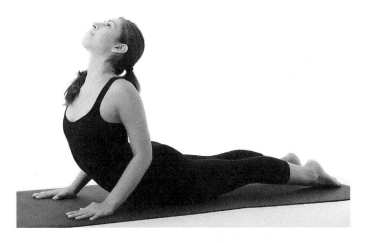

Lying prone with the forehead on the floor, place the palms down by the shoulders and shrug the shoulder blades down the back. Awaken the legs as in Salabhasana, internally rotate the thighs, and press the tailbone toward the heels. Lift the chest as high as possible without using the hands, then pressing the hands down, lift the chest slightly higher with each inhale, staying there with the exhale and drawing the spine forward toward the heart. Continue in this manner, moving breath by breath to the deepest back bend while remaining comfortable. In pressing the palms down, energetically spiral them out (without actually moving them), feeling from this action how the elbows draw slightly in, the chest expands, and the lower tips of the shoulder blades draw in toward to heart.

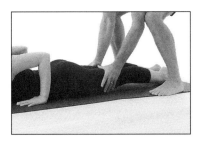

Apply Clasping Rotation on the thighs to cue their internal rotation while pressing the legs together and verbally cueing the student to radiate energetically down through the legs while rooting the feet into the floor so much that the knees lift off the floor.

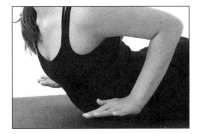

Verbally cue the student to lift the chest as high off the floor as is comfortable without using the hands to leverage the lift at all, and then cue to root the hands onto the floor.

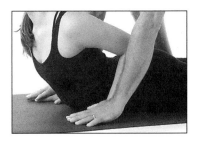

Use Light Hands to cue rooting the hands and creating a feeling of spiraling them outward to help draw the elbows in and open across the chest.

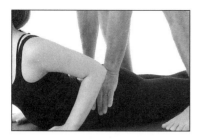 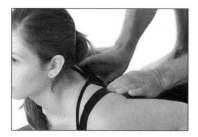 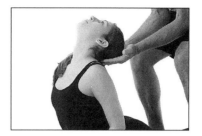

Use Hip Handles with your thumbs to the student's sacrum to cue pressing the tailbone toward the heels, thereby maintaining space in the lower back.

Verbally cue the student to press the hands evenly into the floor to lift slightly higher with each inhalation, holding at that height during the exhalation while lifting the sternum. Apply Finger Draws down the shoulder blades to enhance the feeling of expanding the heart center.

As the student moves breath by breath to the fullest comfortable back bend, use a Light Hand to support the back of the head, if the student feels comfortable releasing the head back.

Modification

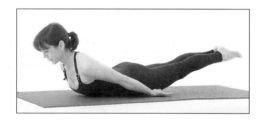

If uncomfortable practicing Bhujangasana, suggest staying with Salabhasana A and B.

Variation

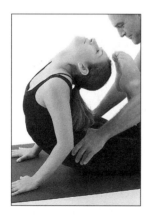

If the student can comfortably release the head back, cue to bend the knees and draw the feet toward or to the head. Do not assist in this; rather, use Hip Handles with Clasping Rotation to help keep the pelvis rooted and to assist in keeping space in the lower back.

Explore Further

Teaching Yoga: page 200

Yoga Sequencing: page 375

Teaching Yoga Resource Center:
  www.markstephensyoga.com/resources

Urdhva Mukha Svanasana (Upward-Facing Dog Pose)

Up Dog is an intense and power-fully awakening back-bending asana. Always offer students the option of Salabhasana B as an alternative in the following conditions: lower-back pain or insufficient arm, shoulder, or leg strength to suspend the body on the hands and feet. In first learning Up Dog, it is helpful to first practice Salabhasana B, which strengthens the lower back and teaches the leg activation that is important in this asana.

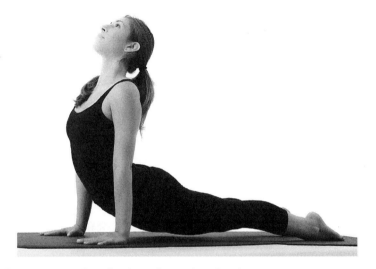

Emphasize active and aligned legs: the feet are extending back and pressing firmly down while the legs are firm, with the inner thighs spiraling up. Encourage students to press the tops of their feet firmly down and create a sense of extending their toes straight back. In rooting the feet down, the legs become more active. From this base in the feet, instruct students to pull their pelvis forward, away from their ankles, press the tailbone back toward the heels, and keep the buttocks soft while allowing the weight of the pelvis to provide traction on the lower back. Do not instruct squeezing the gluteal muscles, which causes the femurs to externally rotate and compresses the sacroiliac joint.

Guide students into the full expression of the asana by asking them to press firmly into their hands, lift their chest, and create a feeling of focusing the back bend in their heart center. Rooting firmly into the knuckles of the index fingers helps to ensure balanced pressure across the hands and wrist joints, thereby reducing the likelihood of strain in the wrists. Strong and balanced rooting of the hands also leads to greater extension of the arms and lifting and spreading of the chest, which is essential in creating the length in the spine required for deepening the back bend. The wrists should be aligned directly beneath the shoulders. If the wrists are positioned forward of the shoulders, students will feel excessive pressure in the lower back; if positioned farther back than the shoulders, they will hyperextend the wrists. Where the shoulders end up relative to the wrists is determined by the movement of the feet in the transition from Chaturanga and the depth of the back bend. Keeping the tiptoes fixed and rolling over them will bring the hips and shoulders farther forward; extending the feet back while pressing the arms straight will result in the shoulders being farther back. There is no correct method. Rather, the unique (and changing) geometry of each student's body— the length of the arms, legs, feet, and torso, plus the degree of their back-bending arc—determines how much to emphasize rolling over the toes versus extending the feet back. Demonstrating these alternatives, highlight the effect on the lower back, wrists, and overall integrity of Urdhva Mukha Svanasana.

Ask students to draw the curve of the back bend up the spine consciously and to create a sense of pulling the lower tips of the shoulder blades in and up as if into their heart center. Students with weak shoulders will tend to hang in their shoulders. This tends to strain the neck, close the heart center, compromise the breath, and exacerbate the tendency to dump into the lower back. Encourage these students to more actively press into their hands (wrists allowing) in order to better draw the shoulders down and away from the ears. The head can be held level; with practice, ease, and stability, the final action of the asana can be releasing the head back. While pressing the palms firmly down, encourage students to energetically spiral the palms out to create more space across the heart center and pull the spine through toward the heart to deepen the back bend.

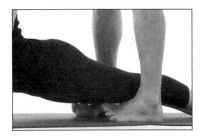

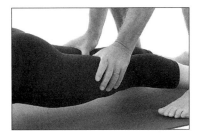

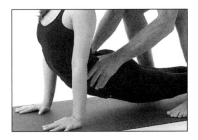

As this asana is generally done dynamically and held only for the pause when filled with breath, the cues need to be given relatively quickly and decisively. As the student draws up into the back bend and you verbally cue firmly rooting out and down through the feet, slide your feet under the mid-thighs and lift your toes into the thighs to emphasize the active engagement of the legs that extends the knees.

Use Light Hands to cue internal rotation of the thighs while verbally cueing the student to strongly press down through the feet and to create a feeling of pulling the hips forward and away from the ankles.

Use Hip Handles and press your thumbs back onto the sacrum to cue posterior rotation of the pelvis, thereby creating more space in the lumbar spine.

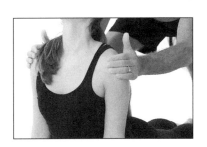

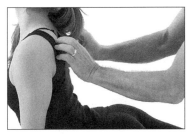

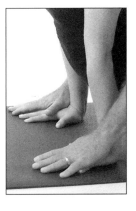

Use very Light Hands to suggest pulling the shoulders back, but do not pull the student's shoulders back, as this can compress the lower back.

Use Finger Draws to cue the shoulder blades down the back while verbally cueing pulling the upper spine forward into the heart.

Placing Light Hands on the student's hands, outwardly spiral your hands while verbally cueing this as an energetic action by the student (without the student actually moving the hands), thereby helping to spread the collarbones and open the heart.

Modification

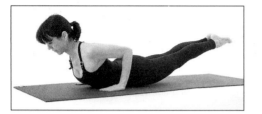

If uncomfortable practicing Bhujangasana, suggest staying with Salabhasana A and B.

Explore Further

Teaching Yoga: page 167

Yoga Sequencing: page 439

Teaching Yoga Resource Center:
www.markstephensyoga.com/resources

Naraviralasana (Sphinx Pose)

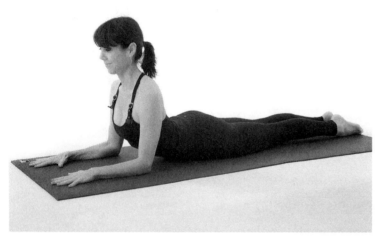

Lying prone, prop up onto the forearms, aligning the elbows under the shoulders and the forearms and hands forward and parallel. Activate the legs as for Salabhasana preparation, rooting the hips and feet, internally rotating the femurs, and pressing the sacrum toward the heels. Rooting the forearms while energetically pulling them back and inward, expand the chest while depressing the shoulder blades and pulling the spine in toward the heart. Over time, lift the head and gaze forward. This is a deceptively deep back bend that can strain the lower back and neck. Reinforce the active engagement of the legs and posterior tilt of the pelvis to maintain space in the lower back. Encourage students to look down to take it easier on the neck.

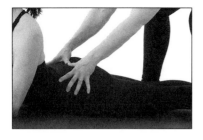

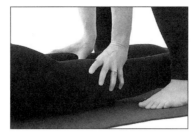

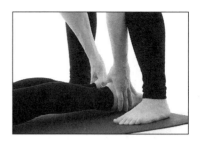

Straddling the student, use Hip Handles with your thumbs turned toward the student's sacrum to cue slight posterior rotation of the pelvis, reducing pressure in the lower back.

Use Clasping Rotation on the student's thighs to cue their internal rotation while also cueing the legs to press together.

Press Light Hands down onto the student's feet to cue their active rooting to the degree that the student's kneecaps lift off the floor, thus awakening the legs.

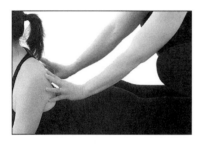

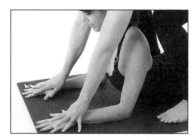

Use strong Finger Draws to cue the shoulder blades down the back while verbally cueing to press the upper thoracic spine into the chest.

With Light Hands on the student's hands, give a cue of sliding the hands back, without them actually moving, to deepen the stretch up through the mid-spine.

Modification

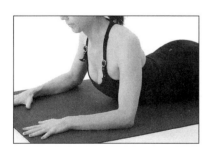

Position the elbows wider apart to back away from the intensity of the back bend.

Explore Further

Teaching Yoga: page 200
Teaching Yoga Resource Center:
    www.markstephensyoga.com/resources

Dhanurasana (Bow Pose)

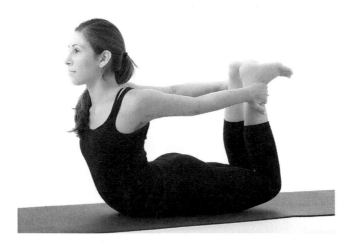

Lying prone, bend the knees and reach back to clasp the ankles. Flex the feet to activate pada bandha and stabilize the knees. Rooting down through the hips, pull on the ankles to leverage the chest and the legs up off the floor, pressing the tailbone back while drawing the spine through toward the heart and spreading across the collarbones. Try to rock back farther onto the thighs to lift the chest higher, then press the feet back up. Focus the back bend in the mid-thoracic spine. If the neck is stable, release the head back toward the feet.

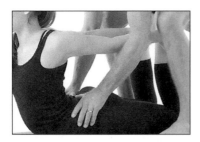

Use Hip Handles to encourage posterior rotation of the pelvis, pressing the sacrum toward the knees.

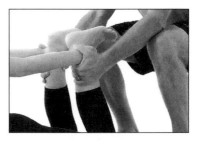

In a low Horse Stance, place your elbows on your knees while clasping your hands around the student's ankles (and hands), then shift your weight gradually back while drawing the student's heels toward your shoulders.

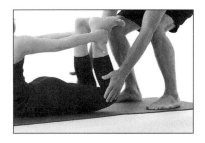

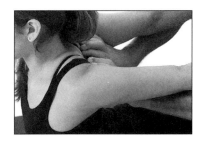

Use Light Hands to cue drawing the knees toward hip distance apart (they will tend to splay out).

Use Light Hands on top of the shoulders or Finger Draws along the shoulder blades to cue drawing the shoulders down and away from the ears.

Modification

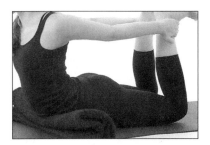

Place a folded blanket under the top front of the student's pelvis (just below the anterior superior iliac spine or ASIS) to ease positioning of the weight of the body farther back and to reduce pressure in the lower back.

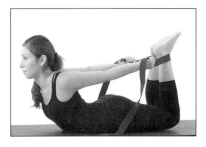

Offer a strap around the feet if the student is unable to easily clasp the ankles.

Variation

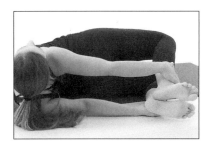

Suggest exploring Parsva Dhanurasana (Side Bow Pose), rolling onto the side of the hip and holding for several breaths before switching sides. Verbally cue students to be aware of pressure in their outer knees (lateral collateral ligaments and menisci).

Explore Further

Teaching Yoga: page 202

Yoga Sequencing: page 378

Teaching Yoga Resource Center:
   www.markstephensyoga.com/resources

Bhekasana (Frog Pose)

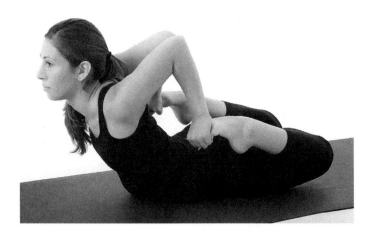

Start as for Salabhasana, then place the forearms on the floor with the elbows under the shoulders as for Naraviralasana. Explore one side at a time, first clasping the right foot with the right hand and drawing the right heel toward the outside of the right hip. In this effort, try to rotate the elbow up and to position the hand on the foot with the fingers pointing the same direction as the toes. Try to rotate the right shoulder forward to square the shoulders toward the front of the mat. If sufficiently flexible, do this with both hands and feet simultaneously. Rooting the hips down and pressing the tailbone back, press the feet toward the floor while lifting the chest (be very sensitive to the knees and lower back). Try to draw the shoulder blades down the back, lower tips of the shoulder blades pressing toward the heart. Gaze down to take it easier on the neck, or forward.

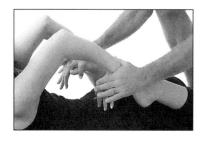 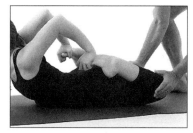 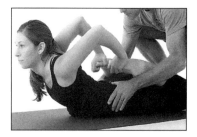

Use Light Hands to assist the student in positioning the hands on top of feet with the fingers pointed the same direction as the toes.

Use very Light Hands to cue the knees into alignment straight back from the hips (they will tend to splay out, potentially straining the outer knees).

Use Hip Handles to cue the posterior rotation of the pelvis, thereby creating more space in the lumber spine while better anchoring the pelvis for the back bend arising from it.

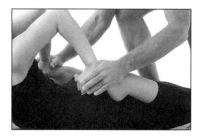 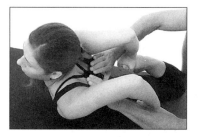 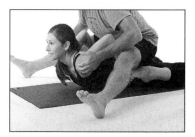

Use very Light Hands to encourage the student to press the feet toward the floor next to the hips while lifting the chest.

Use Finger Draws to encourage drawing the shoulder blades down the back while verbally cueing the lifting of the chest.

If the student can press the feet to the height of the pelvis, sit upright in the preparatory position for Upavista Konasana (Wide-Angle Forward Fold Pose), placing your sitting bones on the sacrum while pressing your legs out and down to further press the student's feet toward the floor. Your hands are now free for upper body cues.

Modification

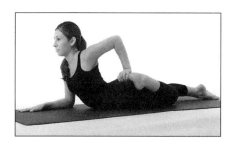

From the Sphinx-like preparatory position, verbally cue and demonstrate drawing the right hand to right foot and holding for several breaths before switching sides.

Explore Further

Teaching Yoga: page 201

Yoga Sequencing: page 374

Teaching Yoga Resource Center:
www.markstephensyoga.com/resources

Ustrasana (Camel Pose)

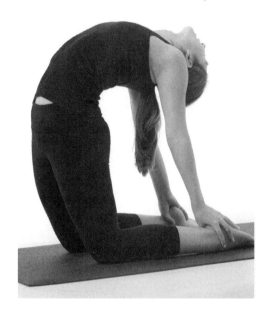

Standing on the knees with the toes curled under (or feet straight back for a deeper back bend) and knees at hip distance apart, place the hands on the hips to press the tailbone down, hips forward, and leverage the lifting of the sternum, creating a feeling of lifting the spine up into the heart. Rooting down through the legs and feet, press the hips forward and the tailbone down while drawing the hands to the heels or ankles (or to blocks). Pressing from the hips through the knees, from the shoulders into the hands, and down through the feet, use these lever points to draw a deeper curve into the thoracic spine while pressing the tailbone down and under and lifting the sternum to the sky.

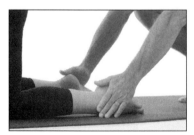

Use Light Hands to assist the student in positioning the feet straight back in alignment with the hips (if pointed back, they will tend to point in).

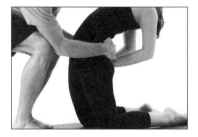

Use Hip Handles around the student's lower back and sacrum to help ease the back into the asana. Use this same positioning to help the student back up.

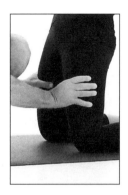

Use Clasping Rotation on the student's thighs to cue their internal rotation.

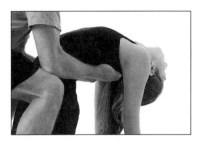

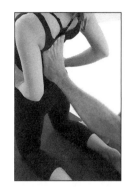

From Horse Stance, use Light Hands under the student's shoulder blades to cue pressing the tips of the shoulder blades as though up into the chest.

Place your heel on the top of the student's sacrum and the ball of your foot against the bottom of the shoulder blades (if your feet are too short for the length of the student's spine, place your other heel on top of your first foot). Then, as the student leans back, your lower heel will press the sacrum down and the ball of your upper foot will press the chest up, thereby creating space on the lower back and across the heart center. Simply press the ball of your foot up along the shoulder blades to ease the student back up.

Modification

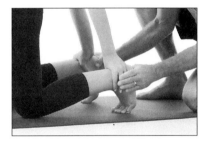

If the student is unable to clasp the heels with the feet in plantar flexion, offer the option of dorsiflexion (with the toes curled under) or place blocks next to the ankles.

Variation

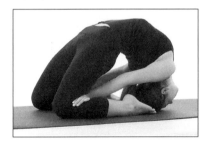

If Ustrasana is easily accessible, explore Laghu Vajrasana (Little Thunderbolt Pose).

Explore Further

Teaching Yoga: page 202

Yoga Sequencing: page 441

Teaching Yoga Resource Center: www.markstephensyoga.com/resources

Laghu Vajrasana (Little Thunderbolt Pose)

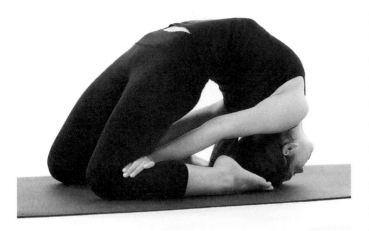

Maintaining all the elements of Ustrasana, bring the hands forward toward or to the knees. Inhaling, release backward, drawing the head toward the floor only as far as the student can, while exhaling, comfortably lift back up to Ustrasana, repeating five times and holding the asana for five to eight breaths on the last drop-back. Maintain the firm rooting of the feet and knees while elongating the spine, being attentive to space and ease in the lower back and neck. Keep the sternum lifting up and the breath steady. Gaze to the third eye.

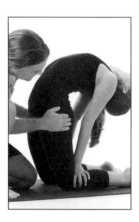

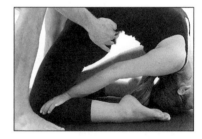

From Ustrasana, verbally cue placing the hands on the ankles or forward as close to the knees as comfortable. Renew the verbal cue (and add Light Hands to accentuate the cue) of grounding down from the hips through the knees (stabilizing) while pressing the feet firmly down (leveraging more space in the lower back).

Standing or kneeling in front of the student, use your hands in a reversed Hip Handles position (fingers around back toward the sacrum) aligned with Finger Spreads to cue space in the lower back and to encourage the hips to press as though forward even as the student reclines back.

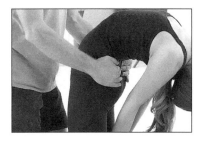

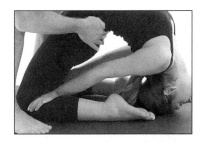

Maintain the same hand position and actions in assisting the student in drawing back up to Ustrasana before again reclining back, repeating several times before holding the student in the more reclined position for up to five breaths. Then assist the student in the same way in coming back up to Ustrasana.

When comfortable releasing the head to the floor, hold for several breaths before coming back up to Ustrasana, or explore Kapotasana.

Explore Further

Teaching Yoga: page 203
Yoga Sequencing: page 395
Teaching Yoga Resource Center:
   www.markstephensyoga.com/resources

Kapotasana (Pigeon Pose)

From standing on the knees, draw the palms together at the heart. Rooting and expanding as for Ustrasana, slowly release back as practiced with Laghu Vajrasana, drawing the crown of the head to the floor. Bring the elbows to the floor and clasp the feet (eventually the knees) with the hands. After five to eight breaths, place the palms on the floor where the elbows were placed, straighten the arms,

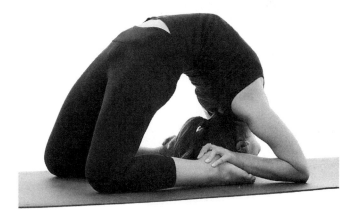

and hold for five to eight breaths. Inhale to come up. Try to maintain the firm rooting of the elbows, feet, and knees, expanding the front of the body while maintaining space and ease in the lower back.

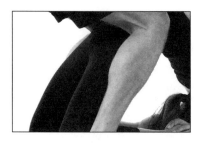 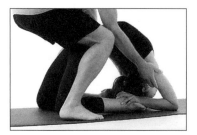 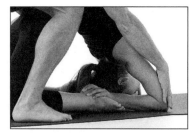

From Laghu Vajrasana, if the student's head reaches the floor, straddle your slightly bent knees around the student's hips to stabilize the hip position, then gradually press your knees back to accentuate the action of pressing the pelvis away from the back.

Maintaining the brace of your knees, use your hands with Clasping Rotation of the student's upper arms to assist their external rotation and flexion as the student draws the hands toward the toes (eventually to the knees).

Use Light hands to encourage the elbows toward the floor.

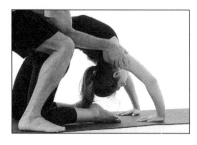 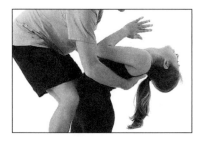

In the first step to releasing, cue the student to place the palms on the floor where the elbows were, fingers pointing toward the feet, then to press the arms straight. Offer Clasping Rotation to assist in externally rotating the upper arms.

Use Light Hands under the mid- and upper-back to assist the student in coming back up to Ustrasana.

Explore Further

Teaching Yoga: page 203

Yoga Sequencing: page 391

Teaching Yoga Resource Center:
www.markstephensyoga.com/resources

Eka Pada Raj Kapotasana II (One-Leg King Pigeon Pose II)

From Adho Mukha Svanasana, bring the right knee just outside the right hand while releasing the left hip and leg to the floor. Prop the left sitting bone as high as necessary to ensure that (a) the sitting bone is firmly supported, (b) the hips are even, and (c) there is no pressure on the inside of the right knee. Keeping the sitting bones grounded and the hips even, clasp the left foot with the left hand (use a strap if necessary), then draw both arms over the head to clasp the foot (or

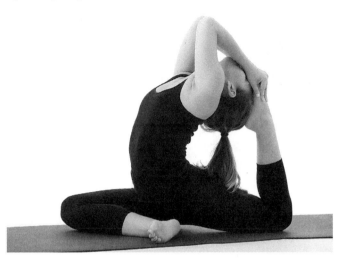

along the strap), and release the top of the head into the arch of the foot. Keeping the hips even and grounded is essential in this asana in order to protect the lower back and front knee. In the back bend, rotate the hip of the back leg forward, internally spiraling that leg to reduce pressure on the sacrum and more easily align the back leg and pelvis. Press the tailbone down while lifting the chest and drawing the elbows toward each other, creating a feeling of lifting the lower tips of the shoulder blades up into the heart while lifting and spreading the heart open toward the sky.

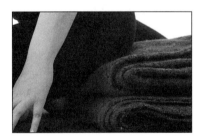

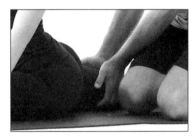

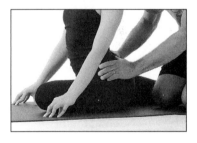

Prop if necessary to ensure that the hips are level and even and the sitting bones firmly rooted, thereby creating the foundation for doing this asana with considerably less risk to the knees and lower back.

Sit in Knees Down position for these cues. In the preparatory position (back leg extended back, fingertips on the floor by the hips), use Clasping Rotation on the back thigh to cue its internal rotation.

Use Hip Handles to cue the pelvis toward a neutral, level, and even position.

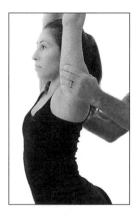

As the student reaches the arms up overhead, use Clasping Rotation on the upper arms to cue their external rotation and further flexion.

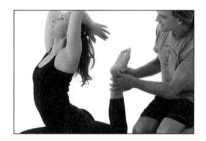

Use a Light Hand to assist the student in bending the back knee, guiding the back foot toward the student's hands.

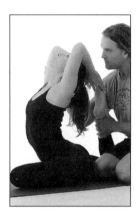

Use Light Hands to assist the student in drawing both hands to the foot while drawing the curve of the back bend farther up the spine and into the heart. Do not offer the popular alternative of one elbow around the foot while clasping the hands overhead, as this brings a twist to the lumbar spine amid a deep back bend, which can severely strain the lower back.

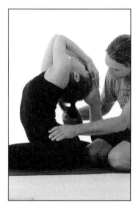

Once the student is in the full form of the asana, use Hip Handles to renew the posterior rotating action of the pelvis, Clasping Rotation on the upper arms for greater external rotation and flexion, and verbally cue releasing the head back toward the arch of the foot.

Modification

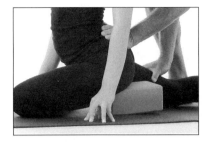

With blocks under the sitting bones, cue staying high up on the fingertips while cueing the alignment and actions in the back leg and pelvis.

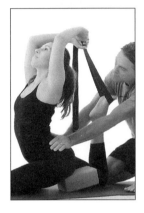

If the student is unable to clasp the foot with both hands, offer a strap from the foot up to the hands. Again, do not offer the popular alternative of one elbow around the foot while clasping the hands overhead, as this brings a twist to the lumbar spine amid a deep back bend, which can severely strain the lower back.

Explore Further

Teaching Yoga: page 206

Yoga Sequencing: page 383

Teaching Yoga Resource Center:
   www.markstephensyoga.com/resources

Supta Virasana (Reclined Hero Pose)

From Virasana (Hero Pose), explore in steps: (1) place the hands a few inches behind the hips, lift the hips slightly to tuck the tailbone under, then sit back down while lifting and expanding across the chest; (2) recline onto the elbows and repeat the actions in step 1; (3) recline onto the back and repeat the actions in step 1.

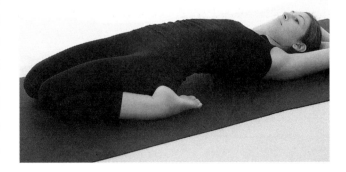

Keep the knees pressing to the floor, thighs rotating internally, tailbone tucking under. For more intensity, draw one knee in toward the shoulder on the same side. Explore drawing the arms overhead and clasping the elbows.

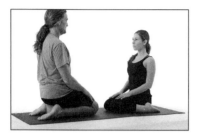

Verbally cue and demonstrate coming into Virasana.

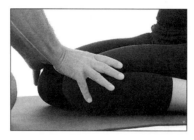

Using Light Hands, press down on the thighs immediately above the knees to reduce pressure on the knees from the pull of the quadriceps muscles.

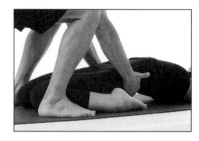

With Open Palms across the lower back and sacrum, press the sacrum under to bring more space to the lower back.

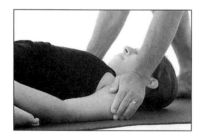

Apply Light Hands to the shoulders, pressing lightly down to expand the heart center.

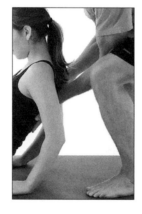

In transitioning up, verbally cue (or assist with Light Hands) first drawing the chin toward the chest to reduce pressure in the neck, then propping up onto the elbows, then hands, then all the way up. If a student is having difficulty coming up, assist with your hands drawing up under the back.

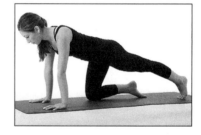

As most students will experience tension in their knees on coming up, verbally cue and demonstrate coming to all fours and extending one leg back with the toes curled under on the floor, then switch sides.

Modification

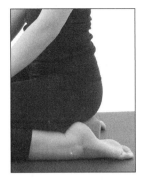

As with Virasana, if a student is unable to sit onto the sitting bones free of strain in the knees or without slumping in the pelvis and spine, offer a block or other bolster to place just under the sitting bones.

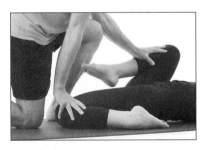

If the student's knees lift off the floor or the student reports tension in the knees or lower back, offer the option of reclining only slightly back onto the hands, or going farther to the elbows. If going to the elbows, offer bolsters to support the back and head.

Variation

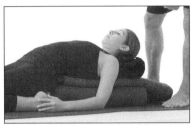

If fully reclined and comfortable yet not feeling a significant stretch through the thighs and hips, cue drawing one knee in toward that shoulder. Place a Light Hand on the front knee and press it down, and place a Light Hand on the top of the other shin just below the knee and press it toward the shoulder.

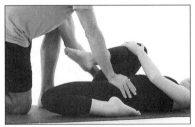

If in the previous position with one knee drawn in, use Hip Handles to orient the hips to be even with each other.

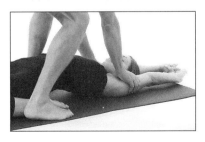

Offer various arms positions to open the shoulders, especially by drawing the arms overhead toward the floor. Apply Light Hands to the lower front ribs to cue them to soften in, then use Clasping Rotation on the upper arms to cue their external rotation.

Explore Further

Teaching Yoga: page 204
Yoga Sequencing: page 429
Teaching Yoga Resource Center:
www.markstephensyoga.com/resources

Setu Bandha Sarvangasana (Bridge Pose)

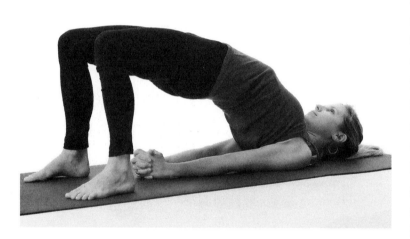

Lying supine, slide the feet in close to the buttocks, hip distance apart and parallel. With completion of the exhalation, feel the lower back press toward the floor and the tailbone curl up. With the inhale, press through the feet (strong pada bandha) to lift the hips up with a feeling of the inner thighs spiraling down, the tailbone leading the way to keep space in the lower back. Interlace the fingers under the back and shrug the shoulders slightly under, just enough to draw any pressure off the neck. Maintaining pada bandha and the internal rotation of the femurs, press down more firmly through the feet to lift the hips. Pressing down through the shoulders, elbows, and wrists, press the tips of the shoulder blades in toward the heart while lifting the sternum toward the chin and spreading broadly across the upper back and collarbones. To release, lift the heel, reach the arms overhead, and slowly roll down one vertebra at a time.

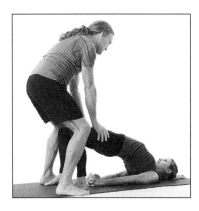

Use Clasping Rotation around the student's thighs to cue their internal rotation and help align the knees with the hips. Play with using your knees against the student's to refine the knee alignment.

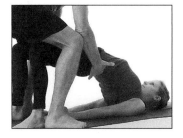

Straddling the student, place Open Palms or Light Hands on the lower back and sacrum to gently lift the pelvis while using moderate pressure to cue a slight tuck to the pelvis, thereby creating more space in the lower back.

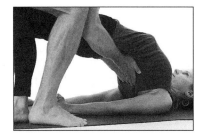

Still straddling (and if tall enough, using your knees to press against the student's outer thighs in support of maintaining their alignment), slide Open Palms fully up onto the shoulder blades, then press your hands up against the student's shoulder blades to cue drawing the curve of the back bends up the spine while lifting the sternum toward the chin.

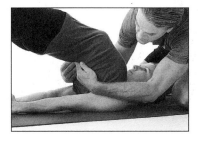

For another approach, sitting in Knees Down Stance overhead from the student, slide your hands between the arms and back to place Open Palms against the shoulder blades and press to expand the back bend into the upper back and heart center. Play with pressing your forearms onto the student's upper arms at the same time to root them down and accentuate the back bend.

Modification

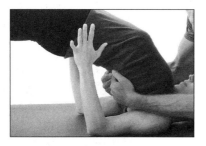

If the student is unable to interlace the fingers under the back and fully extend the arms with the wrists and elbows on the floor, cue bending the elbows and rooting them down into the floor with the forearms and fingers pointing up.

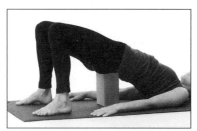

If the basic asana is too much for the student, place a block under the sacrum for a more supported position.

Explore Further

Teaching Yoga: page 204

Yoga Sequencing: page 426

Teaching Yoga Resource Center:
www.markstephensyoga.com/resources

Urdhva Dhanurasana (Upward-Facing Bow Pose or Wheel Pose)

Start as for Setu Bandha Sarvangasana with the feet parallel and close to the hips; place the palms on the floor by and in line with the shoulders. Position the elbows to point straight up by externally rotating the shoulders; if unable to do this, play with separating the hands a little wider and turning the fingertips slightly out to ease the external rotation, creating a feeling of sliding the palms back to root the shoulder blades against the back ribs. With an

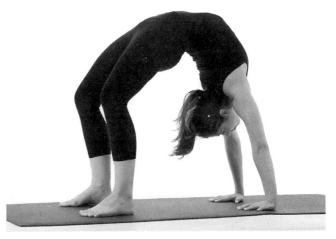

inhalation, press onto the top of the head with the hips lifted off the floor and reaffirm the positioning of the elbows and shoulders. With an inhalation, press the arms straight. Maintain pada bandha, active legs, internal rotation of the femurs, and lengthen the tailbone towards the knees. Press evenly down through the hands, actively externally rotating the arms and expanding across the upper back and chest. Over time, deepen the asana by bringing the hands toward the feet. If the wrists are strained or the elbows slightly bent, explore placing the hands on blocks set against the wall at a forty-five-degree angle.

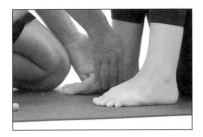

Use Light Hands to help the student position the feet and hands, and Finger Flicks to cue pada bandha.

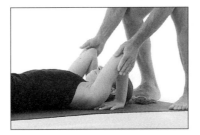

Use Light Hands to cue alignment of the knees with the hips and the elbows with the shoulders (both will tend to splay out).

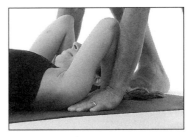

With Light Hands on the student's hands, spiral your hands outward and pull them slightly back to suggest the same energetic actions by the student, thereby helping to maintain alignment of the elbows and root the shoulder blades against the back ribs while moving to the next stage.

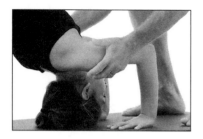 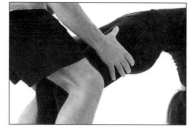 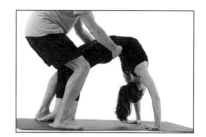

After verbally cueing the student to press onto the top of the head, use Clasping Rotation on the upper arms to assist their external rotation as the student presses the arms straight. Renew this cue once the arms are straight. Never pull the shoulders toward you, and be absolutely clear that you are externally rotating and thereby stabilizing the shoulders, as the opposite rotation or pulling can dislocate the shoulder.

Slightly straddling the student with your knees outside the student's knees, press lightly to help align the knees with the hips while using Clasping Rotation to cue internal rotation of the thighs.

Place Light Hands on the student's lower back and sacrum to gently lift the pelvis while using moderate pressure to cue a slight tuck to the pelvis, thereby creating more space in the lower back. Verbally cue to press the legs straighter and meet the resulting pressure against your hands with equal resistance.

Modification

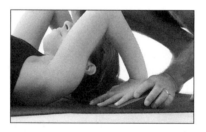

If the student is unable to fully extend the elbows, encourage the student to come down and stay with Setu Bandha Sarvangasana and Dhanurasana until the shoulders and arms open, or explore placing wedges or angled blocks under the hands.

Variation

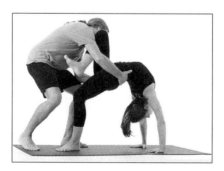

If the student is stable and at ease, verbally cue gradually lifting one foot off the floor, then lifting that knee up and eventually extending the leg straight up into the Eka Pada (One Leg) variation. Use Hip Handles or Light Hands at the back of the pelvis to add stability.

Explore Further

Teaching Yoga: page 205
Yoga Sequencing: page 435
Teaching Yoga Resource Center:
   www.markstephensyoga.com/resources

Viparita Dandasana (Inverted Staff Pose)

Start with the preparatory step of Urdhva Dhanurasana, where the crown of the head is on the floor; draw the elbows to the floor, shoulder distance apart, and interlace the fingers around the head as in Sirsasana I (Headstand I). Pressing firmly down through the forearms, lift the head off the floor, extend the legs straight, draw the feet

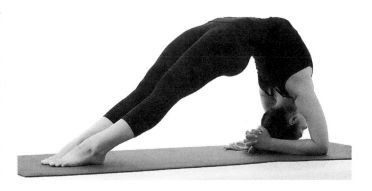

together, and energize down through the legs and feet. Rooting through the forearms and feet, strongly internally rotate the thighs, press the tailbone toward the heels, and expand across the chest.

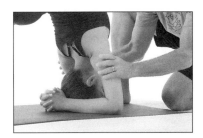

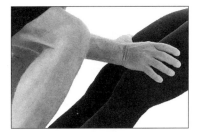

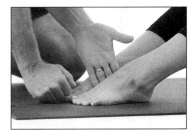

Once the student positions the elbows on the floor, use Clasping Rotation on the upper arms to cue their external rotation while verbally cueing the student to more firmly root down through the forearms, thereby creating more space under the head.

Verbally cue the student to slowly extend the legs, draw the feet together, root the balls of the feet, and internally rotate the thighs while keeping the legs fully extended and awake. Use Clasping Rotation on the mid-thighs to cue their internal rotation.

Use your toes or Light Hands to emphasize rooting the balls of the feet, and use Finger Flicks to emphasize pada bandha.

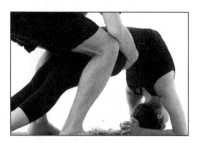

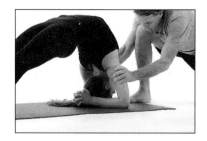

Apply Open Palms to the student's lower back and sacrum, directing the pressure toward the heels to create more space in the lower back.

Use Light Hands to further cue the elbows to stay aligned under the shoulders, and renew the external rotation of the upper arms with Clasping Rotation.

Modification

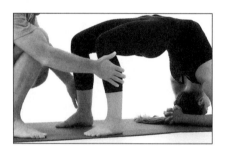

In preparation for the fuller expression of the asana, cue keeping the knees bent and aligned above the heels, hip distance apart.

Variation

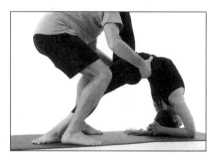

If the student is stable and at ease, verbally cue gradually lifting one foot off the floor, then lifting that knee up and eventually extending the leg straight up into the Eka Pada (One Leg) variation. Use Hip Handles or Light Hands at the back of the pelvis to add stability.

Explore Further

Teaching Yoga: page 206

Yoga Sequencing: page 449

Teaching Yoga Resource Center:
   www.markstephensyoga.com/resources

Natarajasana (King Dancer Pose)

From Tadasana (Mountain Pose), flex the right knee to draw the right foot up toward the right hip. Clasping the right foot with the right hand, rotate the right elbow in and up while extending the right leg back and up from the hip. Lift the left arm overhead, bend the left elbow, and clasp the right foot. Maintain pada bandha in the standing foot to help stabilize the foot and ankle joint. Keep the standing leg straight and strong while aware of the tendency to lock the standing knee. Try to keep the pelvis level to create a symmetrical foundation for the full extension of the spine. Pressing the tailbone back and down, expand the chest, pressing the lower tips of the shoulder blades forward and up to open the heart center. If stable and at ease, release the crown of the head toward the arch of the foot and draw the elbows together. Breathe!

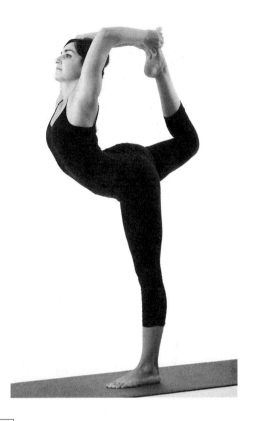

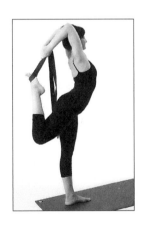

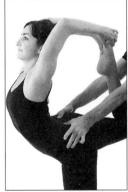

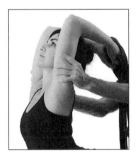

Mirroring the student in Tadasana, verbally cue and demonstrate looping an open strap around the ball of the foot, then bending that knee to draw the heel toward the hip while clasping the strap overhead with both hands.

In Mountain Stance behind the student, use Hip Handles to simultaneously assist with balance and to cue the hips to remain level while using Clasping Rotation to cue the anterior rotation of the pelvis.

Use Clasping Rotation on the upper arms to cue their external rotation and flexion; also use this clasp to suggest lifting the sternum up rather than folding the torso forward as the student brings the hands along the strap to possibly clasp the foot.

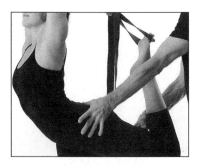

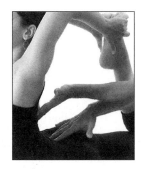

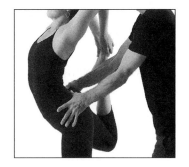

Use an Open Palm on the outer side of the lifted hip to assist stability while using the other hand to cue internal rotation of the lifted leg.

If the student is able to clasp the foot with the hands, use Hip Handles to renew level hips, then use a Light Hand up the mid-spine to cue lifting the chest, thereby drawing the curve up the spine.

In transitioning out, stand slightly to the side of the student and use Light Hands or Hip Handles to ease the student back to standing on both feet.

Modification

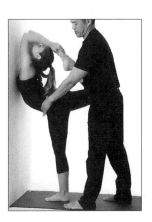

Explore practicing next to a wall for added stability. Play with keeping the chest against the wall to assist in lifting the chest rather than dropping it toward to the floor.

Explore Further

Teaching Yoga: page 207

Yoga Sequencing: page 400

Teaching Yoga Resource Center:
   www.markstephensyoga.com/resources

Matsyasana (Fish Pose)

From Pindasana (Embryo Pose), slowly release the spine to the floor, clasping and pulling on the feet to leverage the chest up and the crown of the head to the floor. Or, from Padmasana (Lotus Pose), recline onto the elbows, clasp and pull on the feet, then ease the head to the floor while lifting the chest toward the sky. Press the knees

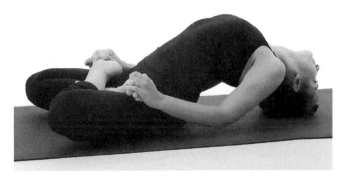

toward the floor while pulling on the feet to deepen the arch through the spine. Transition directly to Uttana Padasana (Extended Leg Pose).

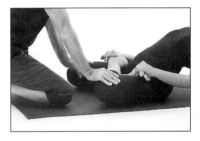

Use Light Hands to press the knees toward the floor. Also squeeze around the inner knees to press the thigh toward the calf, thereby reducing pressure in the knees.

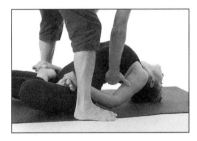

Straddling the student in Horse Stance, place your hands under the shoulder blades to cue lifting the heart toward the sky.

Variation

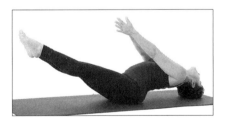

Verbally cue transitioning directly into Uttana Padasana.

Explore Further

Teaching Yoga: page 208

Yoga Sequencing: page 400

Teaching Yoga Resource Center:
www.markstephensyoga.com/resources

Uttana Padasana (Extended Leg Pose or Flying Fish Pose)

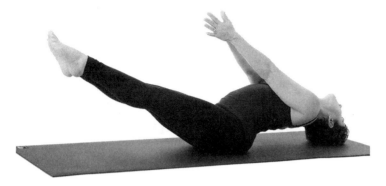

Lying supine, prop up onto the elbows with the fingertips slightly under the buttocks, pressing down through the elbows to press the chest up. Be sensitive to the neck in releasing the head back. For the full asana, lift the legs about a foot off the floor, keeping them straight and strong; release the top of the head to the floor, and draw the palms together over the legs at the same angle as the legs. Internally rotate the thighs, press the tailbone toward the heels, draw the tips of the shoulder blades up into the chest, energize out through the arms and fingertips, and gaze to the tip of the nose.

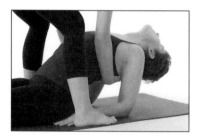

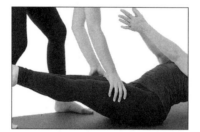

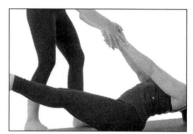

In setting up for the asana, verbally cue the student to slide the hands under the hips while rooting the elbows down and lifting the chest up, then exploring easing the head back. Straddling the student, press Open Palms up against the shoulder blades to accentuate the heart opening stretch across the chest.

If it's okay with the student's neck and lower back, ease the head to the floor while verbally cueing to elevate the legs off the floor. Stepping back, use Light Hands and consider Clasping Rotation on the thighs to cue their internal rotation while verbally cueing the student to strongly radiate out and down through the legs and feet.

Cue the student to press the palms together with straight arms extended forward and up and at the same angle as the legs. Use Light Hands to emphasize pressing the palms firmly together, and verbally cue continuously pressing the upper spine up into the heart center while being sensitive to the neck and lower back.

Modification

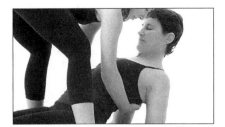

Staying with the prep position, offer the option of tucking the chin toward the chest to prevent hyperextension of the neck.

Explore Further

Teaching Yoga: page 208

Yoga Sequencing: page 442

Teaching Yoga Resource Center:
www.markstephensyoga.com/resources

Chapter 8

Seated and Supine Twists

TWISTS DELIGHTFULLY PENETRATE DEEP INTO THE BODY'S CORE, stimulating and tonifying internal organs, particularly the kidneys and liver, while creating suppleness and freedom in the spine and opening the chest, shoulders, neck, and hips. Active supine twists, such as Jathara Parivartanasana (Revolving Twist Pose), strengthen the abdominal oblique muscles, which are an important muscle group in many asanas involving rotational movement, such as Parsvakonasana (Side Angle Pose) and Astavakrasana (Eight-Angle Pose).

Regular twisting helps maintain the normal length and resilience of the spine's soft tissues and the health of the vertebral disks and facet joints of the spine, restoring the spine's natural range of motion. In a beautiful poetic irony, we find that in twisting our body more and more into a pretzel, we more easily unwind the accumulated physical and emotional tension contained inside. Along with this release of tension, twists tend to bring the bodymind to a more neutral, sattvic state. Thus they are neither generally warming nor cooling, but both: warming if coming from a relatively cool condition, cooling if coming from a relatively warm condition. These qualities allow us to place twists in a variety of places in any given sequence.

Gradually introduce twists throughout the warming part of the practice as well as on the pathway to the peak as a means of reducing tension that may arise in doing asanas from other asana families. The dynamic twisting action of Jathara Parivartanasana is generally warming and can be done as part of relieving tension and maintaining warmth in the body at any time during practice. Releasing the large outer layers of the trunk muscles with forward bends, back bends, and side bends allows easier and fuller rotation at the deep level of the small spinal muscles.

As neutralizing asanas, twists are excellent for calming anxiety and relieving lethargy. Twists will also mildly stimulate the nervous system and reawaken energy following deeply relaxing sequences of forward bends and hip openers. Along with preparatory warming asanas from other asana families, twists are excellent preparation for back bends and excellent initial neutralizing asanas (including calming) following back bends. They are excellent for specifically neutralizing the spine after deep back bends and forward bends, and can be creatively explored in a variety of nontwisting asanas such as Utkatasana (Chair Pose), Virasana (Hero Pose), Gomukhasana (Cow Face Pose) but without its arm component or forward fold, Ardha Prasarita Padottanasana (Half Spread-Leg Forward Fold Pose), and Utthita Hasta Padangusthasana (Extended Hand to Big Toe Pose).

Twists done gently are cooling and should be explored in that way as part of the integrative pathway toward Savasana (Corpse Pose). However, prior to settling into Savasana, follow any twists with a symmetrical forward fold such as Paschimottanasana (West Stretching Pose or Seated Forward Fold) to further release tension in the spine and any sense of imbalance that may have arisen in twisting one side and then the other. Always practice any given twist evenly on each side, promoting balance.

Ardha Matsyendrasana (Half Lord of the Fishes Pose)

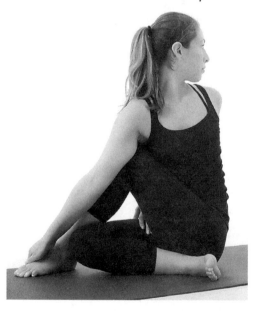

From Dandasana (Staff Pose), slide the feet in halfway and draw the right heel back and under toward the outside of the left hip, then place the left foot on the floor just outside the right knee. Clasp the knee with both hands to leverage the anterior rotation of the pelvis and lengthening of the spine while pressing down through the sitting bones and left foot. Stretch the right arm up to lengthen through the spine and shoulder, then rotate the mid-torso to the left, either clasping the left knee, drawing the right elbow or shoulder across the left knee to leverage the twist, or reaching the right arm along the outside of the lower left leg and clasping the inner left foot.

Keep the sitting bones rooted, and press the right foot down as though trying to stand on it. With each inhale, back slightly out of the twist to more easily elongate the spine, twisting farther with each exhale. Keep the shoulder blades drawing down the back, heart center spacious, and breath steady. Gaze to the left. Advanced students can transition out through Eka Pada Koundinyasana B (One-Leg Sage Koundinya's Pose B) to Chaturanga Dandasana (Four-Limbed Staff Pose).

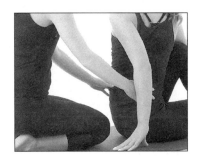

Sitting in Knees Down or Noose Stance, use Hip Handles with Clasping Rotation to emphasize keeping the hips even while rooting down through the sitting bones and rotating the pelvis to neutral.

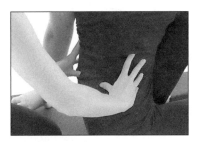

Use Finger Spreads between the top of the pelvis and the lower side ribs to cue lengthening up though the lower back and torso.

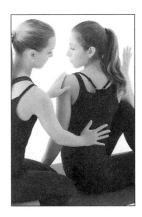

Use Open Palms to encourage the twist: place one palm just beneath the lower back ribs on the side the student is twisting toward, the other palm on the top front of the opposite shoulder. With the student's inhalation, use the lower hand to encourage lifting the rib cage; with the exhalation, use both hands to assist the twist.

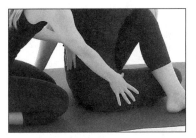

For further refinement, go back to the foundation of the pose and use Clasping Rotation at the top of abducted (lower) thigh to cue its external rotation. Explore using Opposite Rotation for this same cue, the finger cueing the external rotation while the thumb renews emphasis on keeping the pelvis in neutral position by sliding up along the outer area of the sacrum.

Modification

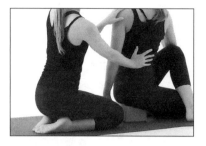

If the student is unable to sit even on the sitting bones (without slumping) or feels pressure in the knees, offer a block or other bolster to place under the sitting bones.

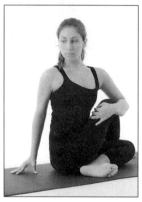

If the student in unable to twist far enough to get the elbow across the knee, cue to clasp around the knee instead.

Explore Further

Teaching Yoga: page 211

Yoga Sequencing: page 367

Teaching Yoga Resource Center:
    www.markstephensyoga.com/resources

Marichyasana C (Sage Marichi's Pose C)

From Dandasana, bring the right heel to the right sitting bone with the knee lifted. Place the right hand on the floor by the right hip, stretch up through the spine and left shoulder and arm, then rotate the torso to the right while drawing the left elbow of the shoulder across the right knee, pressing against the knee to leverage the twist. With more flexibility, reach the left arm around the right 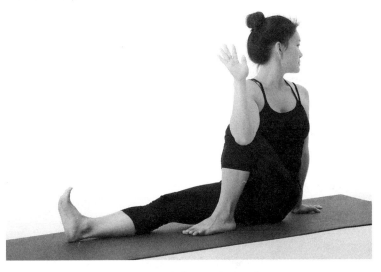 thigh and shin to clasp the right wrist behind the back. Ground down through the sitting bones and extend out through the strongly engaged left leg. With each inhale, back slightly out of the twist to more easily elongate the spine, twisting farther with each exhale. Keep the shoulder blades drawing down the back, heart center spacious, and breath steady. Gaze to the left. Advanced students can transition out through Eka Pada Bakasana (One-Leg Crane Pose) to Chaturanga Dandasana.

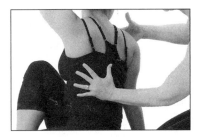

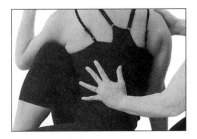

Once the right heel is brought in from Dandasana, verbally cue and demonstrate clasping it with both hands to leverage rotation of the pelvis to neutral and greater extension up through the spine and across the chest, then placing the right hand on the floor by the right hip while stretching the left arm straight up. With Open Palms on both sides of the back side ribs, assist the initial twisting action by continuing to encourage length along the left side while the student draws the left elbow or shoulder across the right knee.

Slide an Open Palm up along the left back side of the torso to encourage greater elongation with the inhalation.

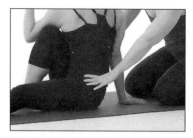

Sitting in Knees Down Stance, use Hip Handles with Clasping Rotation to emphasize keeping the hips even while rooting down through the sitting bones and maintaining the pelvis in its neutral position.

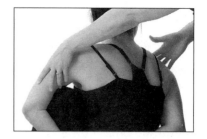

Use Clasping Rotation of the student's upper left arm to assist its internal rotation as the student explores wrapping that arm around the thigh and shin while bringing the opposite arm around behind the back to clasp its wrist.

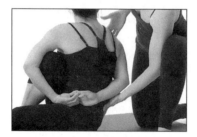

Observing for the tendency to collapse the spine in the effort to wrap and clasp, either verbally cue backing away to a more accessible position or use Open Palms to encourage the twist: place one palm just beneath the lower back ribs on the side the student is twisting toward, and the other palm on the top front of the opposite shoulder. With the student's inhalation, use the lower hand to encourage lifting the rib cage; with the exhalation, use both hands to assist the twist.

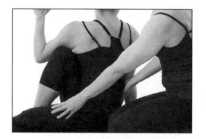

Verbally cue continued grounding of the sitting bones and a strong line of energy out through the extended leg while keeping that foot flexed and that thigh internally rotating to the feet, the knee and toes pointing up. Use Light Hands to cue these qualities of alignment and energetic action.

Modification

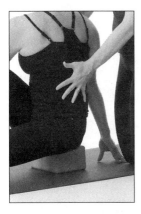

If the student is unable to sit even on the sitting bones (without slumping) or feels pressure in the knees, offer a block or other bolster to place under the sitting bones.

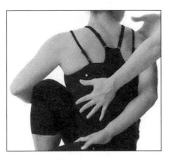

If the student in unable to twist far enough to get the shoulder across the knee, cue to either draw the elbow across the knee or to clasp the hand around the knee instead, keeping the other hand either on the floor to assist elongation of the spine or trying to wrap that arm around the back to clasp the inner left thigh.

Explore Further

Teaching Yoga: page 211

Yoga Sequencing: page 399

Teaching Yoga Resource Center:
   www.markstephensyoga.com/resources

Parivrtta Janu Sirsasana (Revolved Head to Knee Pose)

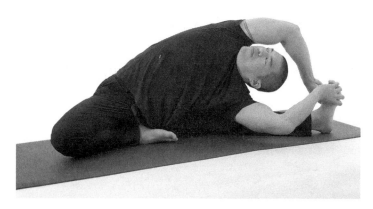

From Dandasana, extend the right leg out as for Upavista Konasana (Wide-Angle Forward Fold Pose) and draw the left heel in as for Baddha Konasana (Bound Angle Pose). Ground the sitting bones, sit tall, firm the right thigh, twist to the left, and lean to the right, moving in stages: (1) the right elbow to the right knee, the left arm down toward the left hip in external rotation, then reach the left arm overhead; (2) the right elbow or shoulder to the right knee or the floor, still rotating the torso open while reaching the left arm over the head to clasp the right foot. If it troubles the neck looking up, either drop the head down or create a headrest with the right hand. Focus on lengthening the spine while in lateral flexion. Make it a side stretch, not a forward bend. If it is easy to clasp the right foot with both hands, use the right hand to press the left thigh out and down, deepening the stretch.

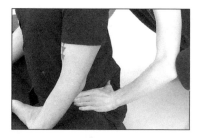

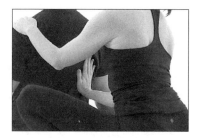

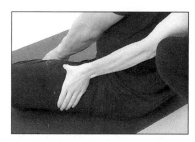

Use Hip Handles with Clasping Rotation to cue pelvic neutrality, if necessary propping up the sitting bones more easily to get the anterior rotation of the pelvis.

Encourage twisting to the left with Open Palms, the right palm on the lower back ribs to cue lifting (on the inhalation) and rotating (on the exhalation), the left hand on the left shoulder to further assist the twisting action.

Apply Clasping Rotation to the left upper thigh or place a knee there to give the same cue (grounding and externally rotating).

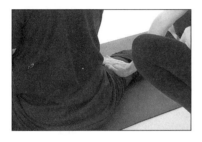 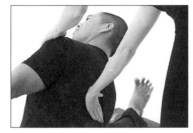 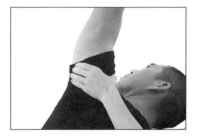

Use Light Hands to clarify the firm engagement of the right quadriceps muscles and to cue the right knee and toes to point straight up (the ankle in strong dorsiflexion).

Reapply Open Palms, now with both hands along the sides of the torso to cue elongation and slight rotation of the torso as the student extends the torso out over the extended right leg.

Use Clasping Rotation on the upper left arm to cue its external rotation, then come back to Open Palms on the sides of the torso to renew the rotation and elongation of the torso.

Modification

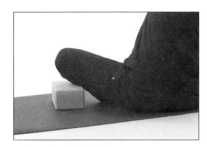

If there is strain in the left knee, hip, or inner thigh, place a block under the knee.

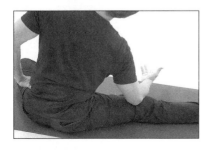

If unable to keep the spine from severely arching into lateral flexion, encourage the student to focus on sitting up tall, twisting to the left, and only slightly leaning to the right.

Variation

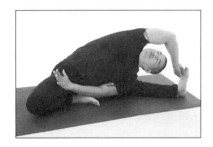

If the student finds it easy to clasp the right foot with both hands, cue placing the right hand on the left upper thigh and pressing it away (in external rotation).

Explore Further

Teaching Yoga: page 213
Yoga Sequencing: page 407
Teaching Yoga Resource Center:
   www.markstephensyoga.com/resources

Swastikasana (Peace Pose)

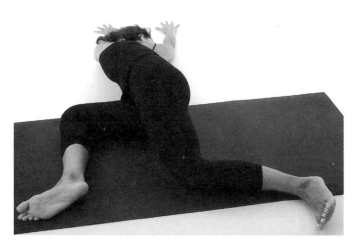

From Dandasana, verbally cue and demonstrate sliding the feet halfway in toward the hips about two feet apart, then release both knees over to the right, positioning the thighs, lower legs, and feet to create a set of right angles before rolling onto the right hip and bringing the hands to the floor to the right. From here, cue students to twist farther around to the right and gradually release their chest to the floor.

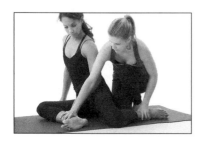

Use Light Hands to help position the student's legs in a set of right angles (at the ankles, knees, and hips).

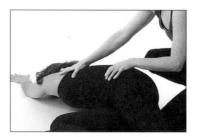

Place a Light Hand on top of the upper hip and on the shoulder blade of that same side, then press the hands away from each other to elongate the torso and slightly deepen the twist.

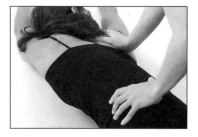

Keeping the Light Hand on top of the upper hip, place the other Light Hand on the opposite shoulder blade, and then press the hands away from each other to further deepen the twist.

Modification

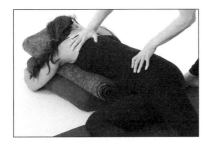

Place a large bolster under the torso to reduce potential strain in the lower back and to create a more restful positioning.

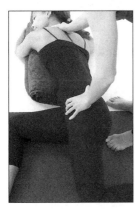

Turn the head in the same direction the knees are pointed to reduce potential strain in the neck.

Variation

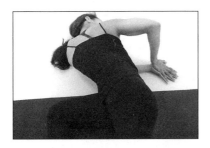

Slide the lower arm farther across and explore creating a prayer twist with palms together and elbows away from each other.

Explore Further

Teaching Yoga: pages 209-10

Yoga Sequencing: page 241

Teaching Yoga Resource Center:
   www.markstephensyoga.com/resources

Bharadvajrasana A (Sage Bharadvaj's Pose A or Simple Noose Pose A)

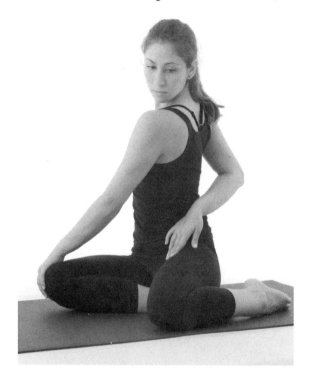

From Dandasana, leaning to the left, bend both knees to draw both heels back to the right, keeping the left ankle under the right thigh. Twisting to the left, reach the left hand behind the back and clasp a piece of clothing, the right inner thigh, or the lotus foot while clasping the left knee with the right hand. Rooting the sitting bones, elongate the spine with each inhale, using the hand clasps to leverage the twist with each exhale. Create a feeling of drawing the upper spine in toward the heart center, drawing the shoulder blades down the back and spreading the collarbones. While twisting the torso to the left, turn the head to the right, drawing the chin slightly down toward the right shoulder.

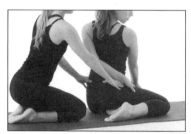

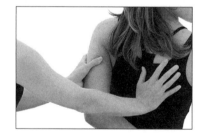

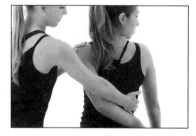

Use Hip Handles with Clasping Rotation to cue rooting the sitting bones along with pelvic neutrality, if necessary propping up the sitting bones to more easily get that anterior rotation of the pelvis.

Use Clasping Rotation on the upper arm that is wrapping to cue its internal rotation, thus easing the positioning of that arm around the back, the student's hand then clasping the right inner thigh or a piece of clothing.

Encourage twisting with Open Palms, the right palm on the lower back ribs to cue lifting (on the inhalation) and rotating (on the exhalation), the left hand on the left shoulder to further assist the twisting action.

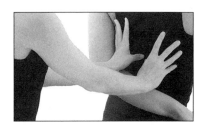

Cue the shoulder blades down against the back ribs using Finger Draws.

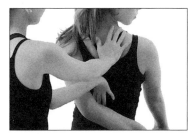

If the student is collapsing the chest, use Light Hands below the shoulder blades to further cue lifting the spine, verbally cueing a feeling of pulling the spine through to the heart while lifting the sternum.

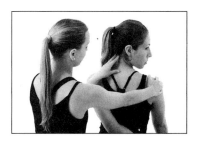

Verbally cue turning the head in the opposite direction of the larger twist, using light Finger Spreads along the back of the neck to cue the chin level with the floor or slightly tucked (sensitive to pressure in the neck).

Modification

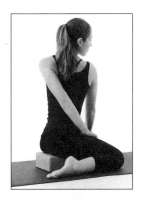

If the student is unable to sit on the top of the sitting bones without slumping, place a block across under both sitting bones.

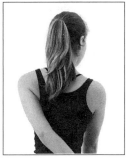

If the student has neck issues, keep the head level and minimize twisting through the neck.

Variation

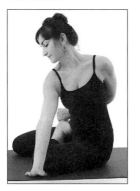

If this asana is easily accessible and the student has healthy knees, explore Bharadvajrasana B (Sage Bharadvaj's Pose B).

Explore Further

Teaching Yoga: page 212

Yoga Sequencing: page 372

Teaching Yoga Resource Center:
  www.markstephensyoga.com/resources

Bharadvajrasana B (Sage Bharadvaj's Pose B or Simple Noose Pose B)

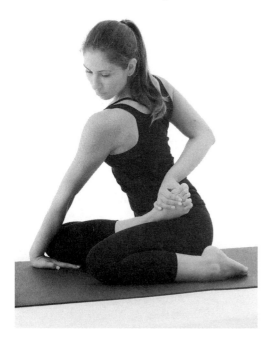

Be very aware of the knees and proceed sensitively. Start as for Bharadvajrasana A, except draw the right heel close to the right hip in Virasana positioning and draw the left foot into half lotus. Twisting to the left, reach the left hand behind the back and clasp a piece of clothing, the right inner thigh, or the lotus foot while clasping the left knee with the right hand. Try to place the left palm on the floor under the left knee and pointing toward the left heel. Rooting the sitting bones, elongate the spine with each inhale, using the hand clasps to leverage the twist with each exhale. Create a feeling of drawing the upper spine in toward the heart center, drawing the shoulder blades down the back and spreading the collarbones. While twisting the torso to the left, turn the head to the right, drawing the chin slightly down toward the right shoulder.

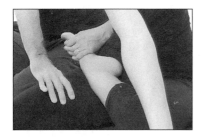

To refine the Virasana positioning of the right leg, use Clasping Rotation to assist the internal rotation of that thigh.

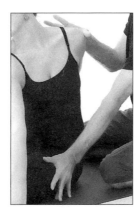

Use Clasping Rotation on the upper left thigh to cue its external rotation in positioning the leg in lotus.

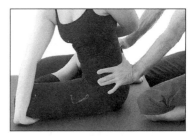

Use Hip Handles with Clasping Rotation to cue rooting the sitting bones along with pelvic neutrality, if necessary propping up the sitting bones to more easily access the anterior rotation of the pelvis.

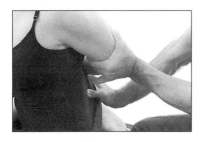

Use Clasping Rotation on the upper left arm to cue its internal rotation, thus easing the positioning of that arm around the back, the student's hand then clasping the lotus foot, the right inner thigh, or a piece of clothing.

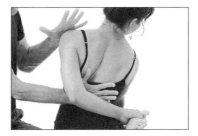

Encourage twisting to the left with Open Palms, the right palm on the lower back ribs to cue lifting (on the inhalation) and rotating (on the exhalation), the left hand on the left shoulder to further assist the twisting action.

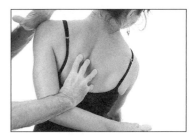

Cue the shoulder blades down against the back ribs using Finger Draws.

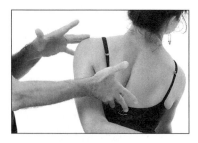

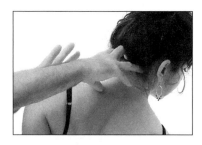

If the student is collapsing the chest, use Light Hands below the shoulder blades to further cue lifting the spine, verbally cueing a feeling of pulling the spine through to the heart while lifting the sternum.

Verbally cue turning the head in the opposite direction of the larger twist, using light finger spreads along the back of the neck to cue the chin level with the floor or slightly tucked (sensitive to pressure in the neck).

Modification

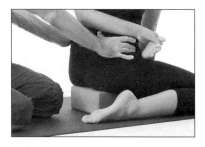

If the student is unable to sit on the top of the sitting bones without slumping, place a block across under both sitting bones. If the student has neck issues, keep the head level and minimize twisting through the neck.

Explore Further

Teaching Yoga: page 212

Yoga Sequencing: page 373

Teaching Yoga Resource Center:
   www.markstephensyoga.com/resources

Supta Parivartanasana (Reclined Revolved Pose)

Lie supine, knees in toward the chest as in Apanasana (Wind-Relieving Pose), arms out, palms down. Gazing over the right hand, release the knee to the left. Alternately, keep the left leg straight out onto the floor and draw the right knee across. The bent-knee position is easier on the lower back. In the held twist, encourage students to be more interested in keeping their shoul-

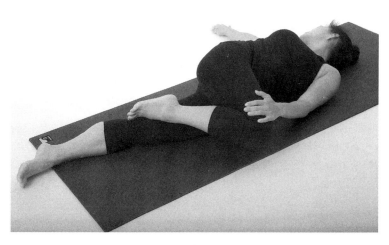

der on the floor than getting the knee to the floor, thereby twisting in the thoracic spine, not the lower back. In the core practice, press the shoulders and palms firmly down while moving the legs, inhaling the legs over, exhaling back to center.

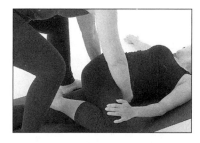

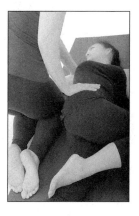

Assist students having difficulty in shifting the lower hip to center by physically lifting and repositioning the pelvis. Do this with bent knees and very aware of your own lower back.

In Knees Down Stance on the opposite side of the student's bent knee, place Open Palms on the top of the upper hip and the shoulder, pressing the hip toward that foot (lengthening, not twisting, through the lower back) while pressing the shoulder lightly to the floor.

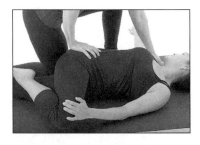

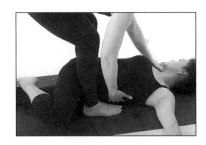

Approach the same basic adjustment in One Knee Down Stance.

For a completely different approach, straddle the student's belly in Mountain Stance, bend your knees to slide your heels back, then lightly yet firmly squeeze your knees together while pressing your calves back against the student's thigh and pelvis while using Open Palms on the torso and shoulder to encourage the twist.

Modification

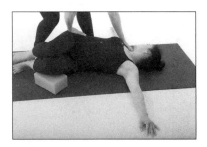

If the student has lower-back issues, cue keeping both knees bent and placing a block under the lower knee and/or between both knees. Use Open Palms to gently encourage the shoulders to the floor.

Variation

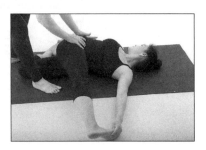

Verbally cue bending the knee of the straight leg and to clasp that foot with the opposite hand while fully extending the other leg and cueing clasping either along it, at the foot, or with a strap around the foot, thereby creating more of a self-adjusting twist and a deep stretch of the tensor fasciae latae and the iliotibial band.

Explore Further

Teaching Yoga: pages 186 and 212

Yoga Sequencing: pages 75-77

Teaching Yoga Resource Center:
www.markstephensyoga.com/resources

Chapter 9

Seated and Supine Forward Bends and Hip Openers

FORWARD BENDS AND HIP OPENERS ARE DEEPLY CALMING ASANAS that draw us into the inner mysteries and dynamics of our lives.[1] The classic seated forward bend (it's also a hip opener), Paschimottanasana, translates from Sanskrit as "West Stretching Pose," signifying the sunset of a practice traditionally initiated facing the rising sun. Here, as we fold into ourselves, the asana naturally lends to deeper self-reflection, which can be emotionally nourishing or difficult, depending on what comes up. Other forward bends like Balasana (Child's Pose) are deeply nurturing; we are in this position during nine months of gestation and naturally return to this fetal position to nurture or protect ourselves.

In stimulating the pelvic and abdominal organs, the subtle energetic effects of forward bends are concentrated in the lower chakras, often revealing base emotions held deep in the body. Holding forward bends for at least a few minutes while refining the flow of the breath allows students to safely explore these feelings. In folding forward we stretch and expose the vulnerable back side of our bodies, most of which we will never directly see. Just as there is often heightened fear in dropping back into the unknown in back bends such as Laghu Vajrasana (Little Thunderbolt Pose), we tend to hold on with the muscles of the back side when folding forward.

To fully release into forward bends, we must let go of an entire chain of muscles that start in the plantar fasciae of the feet and move through the Achilles tendons, gastrocnemii, and solei in the lower legs; hamstrings and adductors on the backs and insides of the thighs; glutei maximi, piriformis, and quadratus lumborum muscles around the back of the pelvis and into the lower back; and then the muscles across the entire back, primarily the spinal erectors, multifidi, and latissimi dorsi (Aldous 2004, 65). This release requires patience as the back side gradually releases and allows the graciousness of the forward bend to manifest. When pursued aggressively, injury to the hamstrings or lower back is likely. Students with disk injuries should explore forward bends with keen awareness and patience, staying with asanas in which they can focus the stretch in the hamstrings and hips, not the lower back, such as Dandasana (Staff Pose) and Supta Padangusthasana (Reclined Big Toe Pose).

While most standing asanas and all forward bends stretch the muscles in and around the pelvis, the purer family of hip openers is found in seated, supine, or prone positions. When stable and open, the hips are the key to our mobility in the world. Yet habitual sitting in chairs and participation in intense athletic activity can combine with genetics to make the hips one of the tightest parts of the body, resulting in limited range of motion and, potentially, strain in the lower back. Open hips are one of the key elements to practicing safe and deep back bends, forward bends, and in sitting effortlessly in Padmasana (Lotus Pose) or another crossed-legged position for meditation.

In exploring hip openers, stay attuned to pressure in the knees; when the pelvis and feet are fixed in position, most positions that stretch hip-related muscles will put pressure in the knees and possibly sprain the knee ligaments or strain muscles attaching in and around the knees. We can develop and maintain a healthy range of motion in the hips through a balanced practice that addresses each of the associated muscles, with a variety of benefits that will show up in standing, back-bending, and forward-bending asanas:

- **hip flexors:** When the primary hip flexors—the iliopsoas and rectus femoris muscles—are tight, the pelvis is pulled into anterior rotation and the lower back tends to develop lordosis. Tight hip flexors also limit back bends. While the standing asanas Anjaneyasana (Low Lunge Pose) and Virabhadrasana I and II (Warrior I and II) are very effective in stretching these muscles, classic hip openers like Supta Virasana (Reclined Hero Pose) and Eka Pada Raj Kapotasana Prep (One-Leg King Pigeon Pose Prep) offer more targeted release of the hip flexors.

- **hip extensors:** Tight hip extensors pull the sitting bones toward the backs of the knees, potentially flattening the lower back and leading to kyphosis in the thoracic spine. Tight hip extensors—especially the hamstrings and lower gluteus maximus fibers—limit forward bending; they are most directly stretched in straight-leg forward bends.

- **hip abductors:** Tight abductors—especially the gluteus medius muscles—are a prime cause of the front knee splaying outward in standing lunge asanas (along with weak adductors), the nemesis of students attempting to cross their knees in Garudasana (Eagle Pose) and Gomukhasana (Cow Face Pose) and a source of pressure on the sacroiliac joint. Again, the asanas in which their tightness most limits the range of motion also most stretch them, especially Gomukhasana.

- **hip adductors:** Tight adductors (along with weak abductors) cause the front knee to splay inward in standing lunge asanas and make it more difficult to bring the legs apart in a variety of standing, arm balance, and seated asanas. (Relatively short femoral heads and/or iliofemoral ligaments will also limit the range of motion, often thought to be caused by tight adductors.) Upavista Konasana (Wide-Angle Forward Fold Pose) and Baddha Konasana (Bound Angle Pose) are the classic seated asanas for opening the adductors.

- **internal rotators:** Tightness in the internal rotators can cause the knees to splay toward each other when standing in Tadasana (Mountain Pose) and limit opening into poses like Padmasana and Virabhadrasana II. Closely associated with the adductors are Upavista Konasana and Baddha Konasana.

- **external rotators:** The most powerful muscles in the body, the glutei maximi are the primary external rotator of the femurs. When tight or overused—as is the case with many dancers—the knees and feet tend to turn out, causing misalignment in many standing asanas and placing pressure on the sacroiliac joint. Gomukhasana and Supta Parivartanasana (Reclined Revolved Pose) effectively stretch these muscles.

Dandasana (Staff Pose)

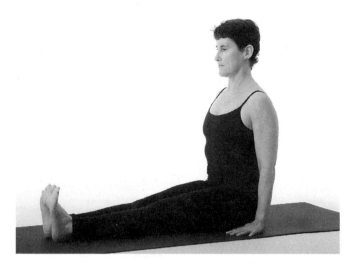

This is the foundational asana for all other seated forward bends. The primary action of all seated forward bends is the firm rooting of the sitting bones. Do not pull the flesh away from the sitting bones, as this will overexpose the hamstring attachments at their most vulnerable place. Sit tall with the legs extended forward, pelvis neutral. If the sacrum tilts back, sit on a bolster to attain pelvic neutrality and neutral spinal extension. Root the sitting bones, flex the feet, firm the thighs without hyperextending the knees, internally rotate the thighs with the pubic bone down and the sacrum slightly in, elongate the spine, shoulder blades down the back, palms rooting, chest spacious, head to the sky.

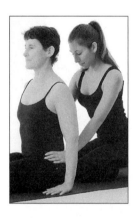

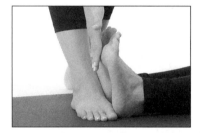

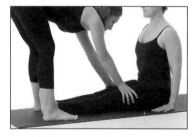

Use Hip Handles to firmly root the sitting bones, and apply Clasping Rotation to guide the pelvis to neutrality.

Simply place your foot across your student's foot to suggest strong lines of energy out through the legs and heels. Also play with using your hands on the students feet to teach dorsiflexion, encouraging greater pressure out through the balls of the feet while drawing the little-toe side of the feet back.

Use Light Hands or Clasping Rotation on the thighs to cue their internal rotation, which should ease the anterior movement of the pelvis.

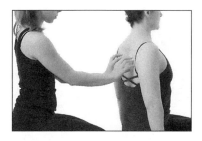

Use Light Hands down from the tops of the shoulders to cue the shoulder blades down the back while verbally cueing the student to lift the sternum while keeping the floating ribs softening in. Also use Finger Draws on the shoulder blades to accentuate this cue.

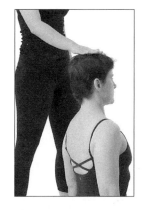

Place a Light Hand on top of the student's head while verbally cueing to more strongly root the sitting bones while sitting as tall as is comfortable.

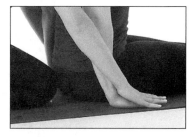

Apply Light Hands to the top of the student's hands to encourage more actively rooting the palms into the floor.

Modification

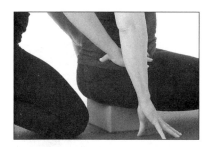

If the student in unable to sit tall with the weight to the front of the sitting bones (pelvic neutrality), offer a block or other bolster to elevate the sitting bones.

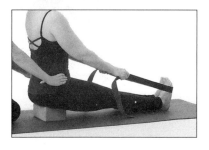

Offer a strap around the student's feet to clasp and pull as a source of leveraged extension out through the legs, the pelvis more forward, the spine taller, and the heart center more spacious.

Explore Further

Teaching Yoga: page 218

Yoga Sequencing: page 378

Teaching Yoga Resource Center: www.markstephensyoga.com/resources

---

Paschimottanasana (West Stretching Pose or Seated Forward Fold)

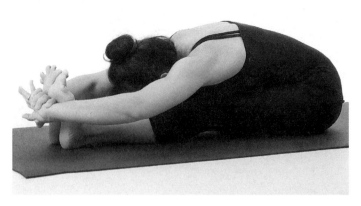

Sitting tall in Dandasana, bring the hands toward the feet as far as possible without bending the spine. Clasp there (or a strap around the feet) to leverage the activation of the legs, lengthening of the spine, and anterior rotation of the pelvis. Draw the torso forward over the legs by rotating the pelvis forward. Stretch the elbows out away from each other, drawing the shoulder blades down the back. Renew the firm grounding of the sitting bones. With each inhale, lengthen the spine; with each exhale, release the torso forward. Be more interested in drawing the heart center up and forward than getting the face to the legs. Keep the legs active, patiently allowing the back of the body to release.

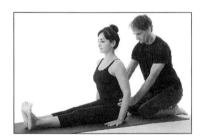
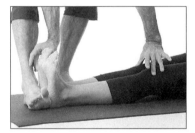
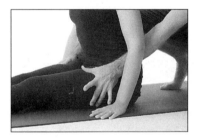

Starting in Dandasana, use Hip Handles to firmly root the sitting bones, and apply Clasping Rotation to encourage anterior rotation of the pelvis to neutrality. Appreciate that for many students the postural form of Dandasana *is* Paschimottanasana; their difference is only in the intention to rotate the pelvis farther forward.

Place your foot against the student's heels to encourage engagement of the legs, and use Light Hands to orient the toes and knees to point straight up.

Verbally cue the student to root the sitting bones while radiating energetically out through the legs and heels, also cueing to keep the legs strongly engaged. Use Light Hands to cue the slight internal rotation of the thighs.

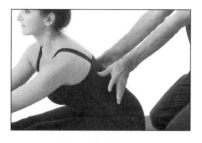

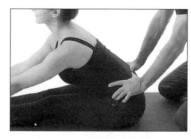

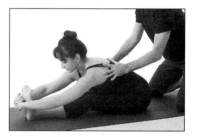

Verbally cue the student to clasp the sides of the legs or the feet and to use the clasp to leverage the greater activation of the legs and upward extension of the spine and torso. Apply Finger Spreads below the side and back ribs or Light Hands up the back to further cue this elongation.

Reapply Hip Handles with Clasping Rotation to now cue the further forward rotation of the pelvis while verbally cueing to keep the spine in its natural form, using clasps along the sides of the legs or feet to leverage the sternum up even while folding forward.

If the student can rotate the pelvis to bring the torso to forty-five degrees, verbally cue to begin folding through the spine with each exhalation, with the inhalation rising back toward the forty-five-degree angle to renew the lengthening of the spine and expansion of the heart center, continuing to move in this dynamic way with smaller and small movements. As the student inhales slightly up, apply an Opposite Rotation cue along the side ribs just below the apex of the curve in the spine to further convey the action of drawing the spine long even while folding forward.

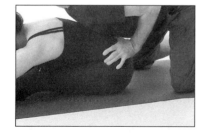

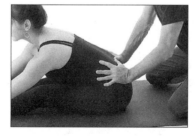

Depending on your relationship with the student, consider placing your sternum against the back a few inches below the apex of the curve in the spine and sliding your sternum slightly up the spine as the student inhales, the pressing more forward on the exhale. This is best done while maintaining Hip Handles with Clasping Rotation, or reach forward to clasp the outsides of the student's feet.

Reapply Hip Handles with strong Clasping Rotation as you verbally cue the student to rise up from the forward fold on an inhalation, posteriorly rotating the pelvis to ease the transition up.

Modification

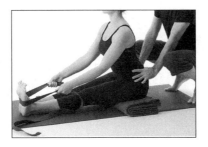

If the student is unable to sit up in the preparatory (Dandasana) form, offer a block or other bolster to place under the sitting bones and a strap to place around the feet (or cue to clasp along the legs), cueing to pull with the hands to leverage the pelvis forward and the spine taller.

Explore Further

Teaching Yoga: page 219

Yoga Sequencing: page 413

Teaching Yoga Resource Center:
  www.markstephensyoga.com/resources

Janu Sirsasana (Head to Knee Pose)

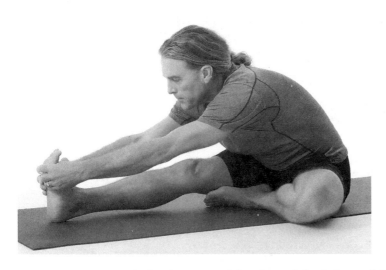

Sitting tall in Dandasana, draw the left heel to the inner right thigh close to the pelvis with the knee resting on the floor or a block. Keeping the sitting bones even and firmly grounded, turn the torso slightly to point the sternum toward the right foot. In folding forward, proceed as for Paschimottanasana while lifting the belly and drawing it slightly toward the right thigh. Renew the firm grounding of the sitting bones and firming of the left quadriceps. With each inhalation, lift the chest slightly to more fully extend the spine. With each exhalation, settle more deeply into the asana.

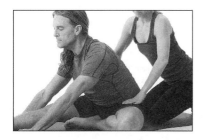 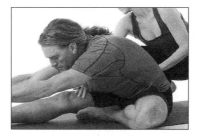 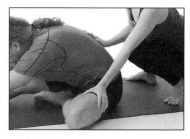

Use Hip Handles to firmly root the sitting bones, and apply Clasping Rotation to encourage the anterior rotation of the pelvis, communicating with the student about any pressure in the bent knee.

Apply a Light Hand to the mid-thigh of the extended leg to clarify its engagement while verbally cueing the student to dorsiflex that foot and energize out through that leg.

Apply Clasping Rotation to the upper thigh of the bent leg to accentuate its external rotation.

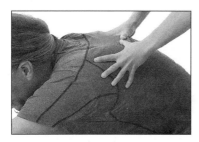 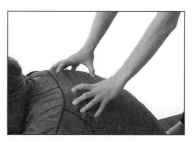

With your hands open wide on the student's shoulder blades, thumbs pointing in, apply Opposite Rotation with your fingers sliding forward and thumbs sliding down while verbally cueing the student to lift the sternum up and forward to lengthen the spine and keep the chest from collapsing.

Use Finger Draws to further cue the shoulder blades down the back.

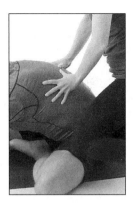

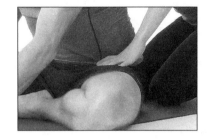

Place your knee on the outer part of the student's bent upper leg to cue its external rotation while either using Clasping Rotation to cue the pelvis to rotate forward or applying Open Palms along the sides of the rib cage to cue lifting the lengthening the torso forward.

Reapply Hip Handles with strong Clasping Rotation as you verbally cue the student to rise up from the forward fold on an inhalation, posteriorly rotating the pelvis to ease the transition up.

Modification

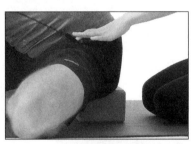

If the student is unable to sit fully up on the sitting bones without slumping, offer a block or other bolster to place the sitting bones.

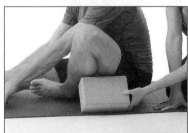

If the student reports tension in the bent knee, offer a block to place under it.

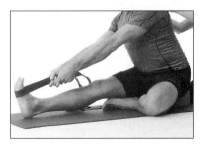

If the student is unable to fold forward without slumping, offer a strap around the foot and cue to pull lightly on it to help leverage the anterior rotation of the pelvis and the lifting of the torso and sternum while drawing the shoulder blades down the back and expanding across the chest.

Explore Further

Teaching Yoga: page 213

Yoga Sequencing: page 407

Teaching Yoga Resource Center:
www.markstephensyoga.com/resources

Marichyasana A (Sage Marichi's Pose A)

Sitting tall in Dandasana, draw the right heel in toward the right sitting bone. Place the left hand on the floor by the left hip and lean the torso slightly to the left while stretching the right arm up. Hinging from the hips, slowly stretch the torso and right arm forward, and wrap the right arm low around the right shin while drawing the left hand around behind the back to clasp the right wrist.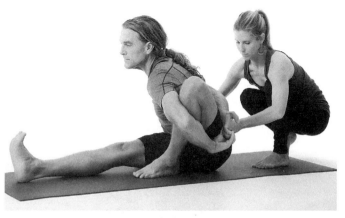

Inhaling, lift the spine and chest; exhaling, fold forward. Press down into the right foot as though trying to stand up on it. With each inhalation, lift the chest slightly to more fully extend the spine. With each exhalation, settle more deeply into the asana.

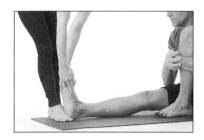

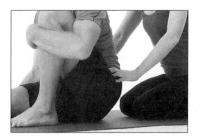

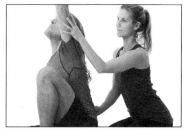

Place your foot against the student's extended heel to encourage the student to press out through that heel, and use a Light Hand to orient the left toes and knee to point straight up, further cueing this alignment by lightly internally rotating that thigh.

Use Hip Handles to firmly root the sitting bones, and apply Clasping Rotation to encourage anterior rotation of the pelvis.

Verbally cueing the student to reach the arm up toward the sky, encourage greater length through that side, shoulder, and arm by sliding a Light Hand up that side and shoulder.

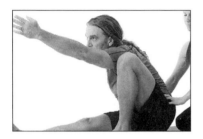 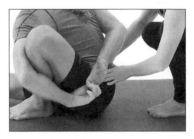 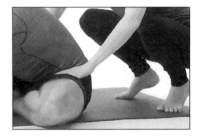

As the student reaches forward to draw the arm around the bent knee, reapply Hip Handles with Clasping Rotation to cue to sustained grounding of the sitting bones and maximum anterior rotation of the pelvis as the source of the forward fold (rather than first rounding the spine).

Once the student clasps the hands behind the back, further apply Hip Handles and Clasping Rotation as before while verbally cueing to lift up through the spine on an inhalation.

Reapply Hip Handles with strong Clasping Rotation as you verbally cue the student to rise up from the forward fold on an inhalation, posteriorly rotating the pelvis to ease the transition up.

Modification

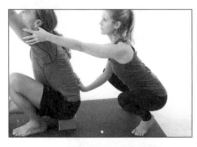

If the student is unable to sit fully up on the sitting bones without slumping, offer a block or other bolster to place under the sitting bones.

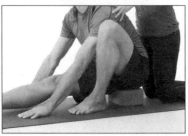

If the student is unable to wrap and clasp the hands, cue either keeping the hands on floor while energetically grounding the sitting bones, sitting tall, and attempting further forward rotation of the pelvis, or making the same effort clasping a strap around the foot.

Explore Further

Teaching Yoga: page 220

Yoga Sequencing: page 394

Teaching Yoga Resource Center: www.markstephensyoga.com/resources

---

Akarna Dhanurasana (Shooting Bow Pose)

Preparing as for Marichyasana A, with one foot drawn in close to the sitting bone, clasp both big toes while rooting the sitting bones and lifting the spine. Slowly lift the foot of the bent leg and draw it back toward the ear. Emphasize the Dandasana elements: active extended leg, anterior rotation of the pelvis, extended spine, open heart center, and steady breath.

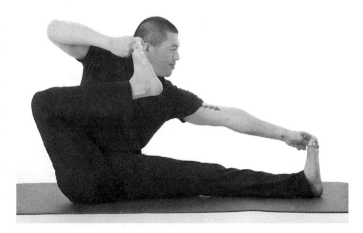

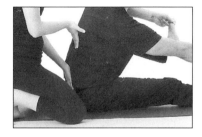

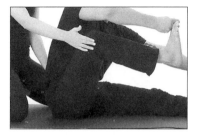

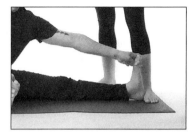

In lifting up the foot of the bent leg, the tendency is to slump. Press an open palm onto the student's sacrum to cue the pelvis forward while sliding a Light Hand up the back to encourage the lift through the torso.

Keeping the Open Palm on the student's sacrum, apply a Light Hand to the lifted knee to encourage the knee toward the shoulder or ear (as it will tend to splay out).

Place your foot against the student's heel and verbally cue energizing out through the leg while flexing the foot.

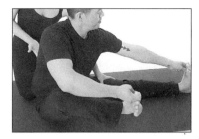

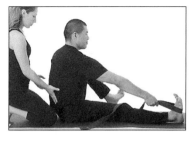

Press an Open Palm onto the student's thigh to encourage its grounding while using your other hand to continue cueing the student's pelvis forward and spine tall.

Use Finger Draws or Light Hands down from the student's shoulders to cue the shoulders away from the ears.

Modification

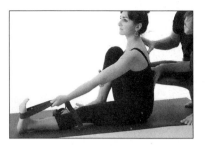

If the student is unable to keep from slumping, offer a strap around the foot of the extended leg and suggest clasping the knee rather than the big toe of the bent leg.

Explore Further

Teaching Yoga: page 226

Yoga Sequencing: page 362

Teaching Yoga Resource Center:
   www.markstephensyoga.com/resources

Balasana (Child's Pose)

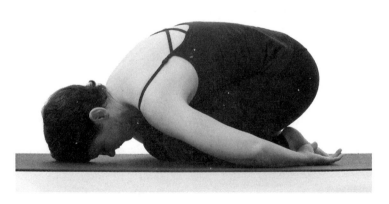

From all fours, release the hips back toward or to the heels, draping the arms onto the floor along the sides of the legs. Bringing the knees wider apart creates an easier release through the hips, easing pressure in the lower back and the knees. Among the most relaxing asanas, Balasana is a place of rest and inner calm. Encourage students to stay with the breath while completely letting go and relaxing deep inside.

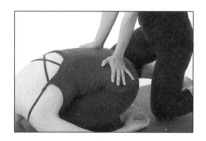

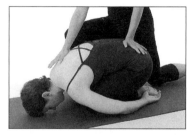

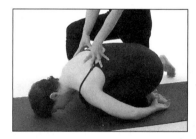

Apply Open Palms to the student's sacrum, sliding your hands down and out to reduce pressure on the sacroiliac joint.

Place one Open Palm just above one side of the student's pelvis and the other Open Palm just below the opposite should blades, then press your hands away from each other.

Apply Finger Draws on the student's shoulder blades to cue more space around the neck.

Modification

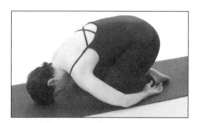

If the student's hips don't reach the heels, suggest separating the knees to more easily release through the hips and thereby relieve pressure from the lower back and knees.

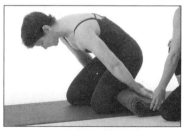

If a student reports tension in the knees, try the knees-apart position; also explore placing a folded blanket (not more than a few inches thick) behind the knees.

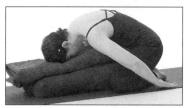

If a student with knees apart is able to fold fully forward, offer a stack of bolsters on the lap to rest over.

Explore Further

Teaching Yoga: page 217

Yoga Sequencing: page 372

Teaching Yoga Resource Center: www.markstephensyoga.com/resources

Virasana (Hero Pose)

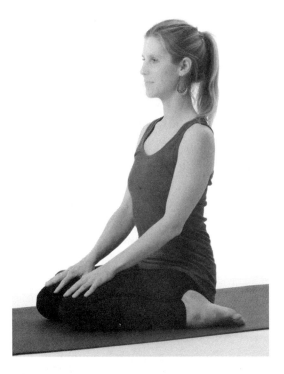

Standing on the knees with the feet extended back, press the thumbs into the middle of the calf muscles behind the knees. Slide the thumbs down the middle of the muscles, spreading them out from the center while drawing the sitting bones to the floor between the heels (or onto a block or bolster). Clasp the knees, root the sitting bones, internally rotate the femurs, and anteriorly rotate the pelvis to neutral while drawing tall through the spine, shoulder blades down the back, and chest spacious. Keeping the sitting bones rooted, with each exhalation renew the light lifting of the perineum, cultivating mula bandha while energizing up through the spine. Allow the head to float on top of the spine, breathing deeply and steadily. This is an excellent asana for all pranayama practices.

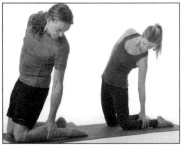

Verbally cue and demonstrate standing on the knees and pressing the thumb tips down the centers of the calf muscles while sitting down between the heels to ease pressure in the knees. Do not press the calf muscles out to the sides, as this introduces a twist into the knees.

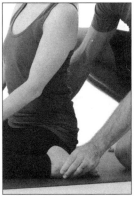

Use Light Hands to assist the student in pointing the feet straight back.

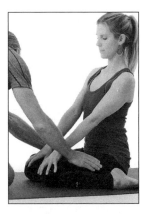

Use Clasping Rotation on the thighs to assist with their internal rotation.

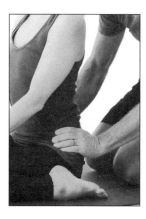

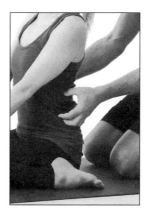

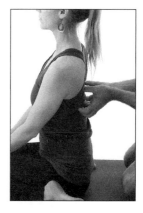

Use Hip Handles to root the hips down and guide the student to pelvic neutrality.

Apply Finger Spreads to the space just below the side ribs to encourage the student to draw up tall through the spine.

Use Finger Draws at the lower part of the shoulder blades to cue the shoulder blades down the back while verbally cueing the student to keep the floating ribs softening in.

Modification

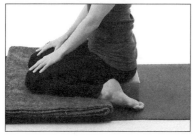

If the student is uncomfortable with the feet in plantar flexion (or unable to fully plantar flex the feet), place a blanket under the shins with the ankles at the edge and the feet resting on the mat.

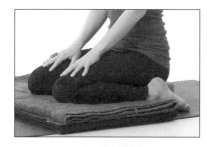

If the student feels pressure in the knees, slumps, or is unable to bring the weight to the front of the sitting bones, offer a block to place between the heels.

Explore Further

Teaching Yoga: page 223

Yoga Sequencing: page 453

Teaching Yoga Resource Center:
   www.markstephensyoga.com/resources

Tiriang Mukha Eka Pada Paschimottanasana
(Three Limbs Facing One Foot West Stretching Pose)

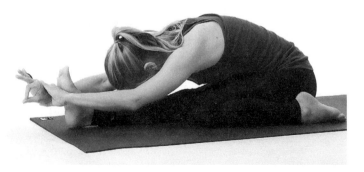

From Dandasana, lean to the left to more easily fold the right leg into the Virasana position. Try to root the sitting bones equally. Fold forward as for Janu Sirsasana. Try to root the right sitting bone more firmly, internally rotating the right thigh while rotating the pelvis forward as the source of the forward fold.

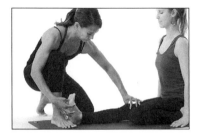

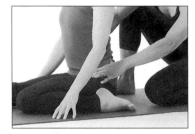

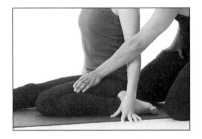

Place your foot against the student's left heel to encourage the student to press out through that heel, and use a Light Hand to orient the left toes and knee to point straight up, further cueing this alignment by lightly internally rotating that thigh.

Use Hip Handles to firmly root the sitting bones, and apply Clasping Rotation to encourage anterior rotation of the pelvis while verbally cueing the student to orient the sternum toward the left foot (not directly forward).

Apply Clasping rotation to the thigh of the bent leg to cue its internal rotation.

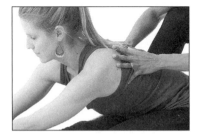

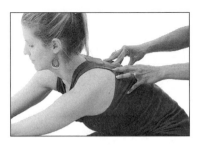

With your hands open wide on the student's shoulder blades, thumbs pointing in, apply Opposite Rotation with your fingers sliding forward and thumbs sliding down while verbally cueing the student to lift the sternum up and forward to lengthen the spine and keep the chest from collapsing.

Use Finger Draws to further cue the shoulder blades down the back.

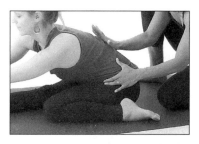

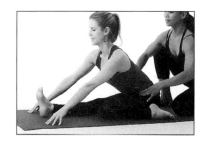

With a Hip Handle pressing down on the Virasana hip, slide an Open Palm up along the student's back, starting well below the apex of the curve in the spine.

Reapply Hip Handles with strong Clasping Rotation as you verbally cue the student to rise up from the forward fold on an inhalation, posteriorly rotating the pelvis to ease the transition up.

Modification

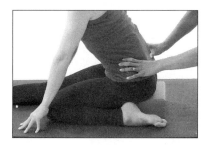

If the student is unable to sit fully up on the sitting bones without slumping, offer a block or other bolster to place under the sitting bones.

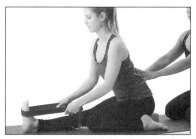

If the student is unable to clasp the left foot with the hands without folding the spine, offer a strap to place around the foot.

Variation

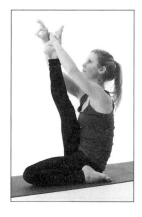

Transition directly from this asana into Krounchasana (Heron Pose).

Explore Further

Yoga Sequencing: page 431

Teaching Yoga Resource Center: www.markstephensyoga.com/resources

---

Upavista Konasana (Wide-Angle Forward Fold Pose)

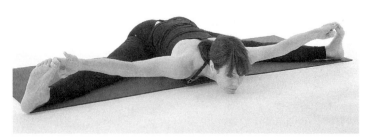

From Dandasana, extend both legs out in abduction. Prop as needed to find pelvic neutrality. Point the toes and kneecaps straight up while firming the thighs, elongating the spine, and spreading across the heart center. Press the hands into the floor behind the hips to help rotate the pelvis forward. If able to sit tall on the sitting bones with the hands off the floor, reach the arms forward and use the hands on the floor to help draw the torso forward. Keeping the sitting bones rooted, legs active, and kneecaps pointing up, move with the breath to fold forward through the anterior rotation of the pelvis, eventually bringing the chest to the floor and clasping the feet. Be more interested in a long spine and open heart than folding down. Gaze either down or to the horizon.

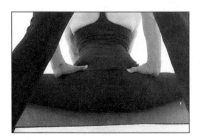

With the student sitting tall in the preparatory position, use Hip Handles with Clasping Rotation to ground the sitting bones and encourage rotation of the pelvis forward.

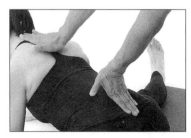

As the student begins to move forward, he or she may tend to slump. Verbally cue to keep lifting the sternum while using a Light Hand up the mid-back and another from the top of one shoulder down to add a tactile cue.

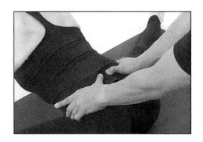

Using Clasping Rotation on the student's upper thighs, and if your hands are large enough, bring your thumbs as close to the sacrum as you can and slide them up the sacrum while your hands are cueing the thighs to stay in position. The Clasping Rotation becomes an Opposite Rotation.

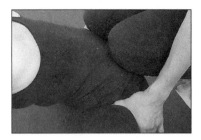

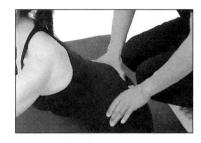

With your hands in Clasping Rotation position on the student's upper thighs, come into Knees Up Stance and slide your knees up along the sides of the spine (without touching the spine) to further encourage anterior rotation of the pelvis and space in the lower back.

As the student inhales to come up, use Hip Handles with your thumbs sliding down the sacrum to help ease the student up to sitting tall.

Modification

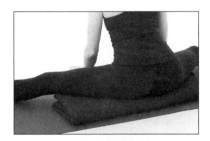

If the student is unable to sit tall on the sitting bones, offer a block or other bolster.

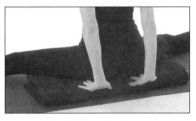

If a student is able to sit tall but can't rotate the pelvis forward, verbally cue to place the hands behind on the floor to assist in lifting through the spine while trying to rotate the pelvis forward.

Variation

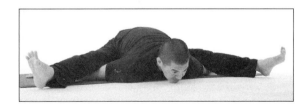

When Upavista Konasana become fully accessible, introduce the student to Kurmasana (Tortoise Pose).

Explore Further

Teaching Yoga: page 220
Yoga Sequencing: page 434
Teaching Yoga Resource Center:
   www.markstephensyoga.com/resources

Kurmasana (Tortoise Pose)

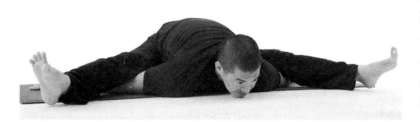

From Upavista Konasana, bring the legs slightly closer together, lifting the knees to create space for extending the arms straight out under the knees. Try to bring the legs closer together, eventually to the shoulders. Grounding the sitting bones, press the legs straight, toes spreading, gaze forward to the horizon. Focus on grounding the sitting bones and extending through the legs and spine. Eventually cross the legs over behind the back and press up to Dwi Pada Sirsasana (Two Legs behind Head Pose), transitioning out through Tittibhasana (Firefly Pose), Bakasana (Crane Pose), and Chaturanga Dandasana (Four-Limbed Staff Pose).

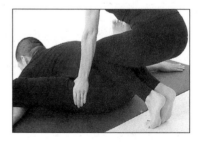

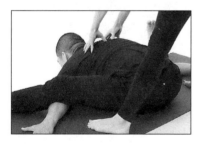

Standing on the balls of your feet in Knees Up Stance, use Clasping Rotation to maintain neutral rotation of the student's thighs while sliding your knees slowly up the quadratus lumborum muscles, from just above the pelvis to the lower back ribs.

Apply Finger Draws to the student's shoulder blades while verbally cueing lifting the chest and drawing the sternum forward toward the horizon.

Modification

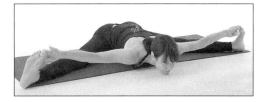

Rather than modifying Kurmasana, if it is inaccessible, keep practicing Upavista Konasana.

Explore Further

Teaching Yoga: page 221

Yoga Sequencing: page 394

Teaching Yoga Resource Center:
   www.markstephensyoga.com/resources

Baddha Konasana (Bound Angle Pose or Cobbler's Pose)

From the preparatory position for Upavista Konasana, bend the knees to bring the feet together. Reduce knee strain by placing a block under the knee or under both knees. Press the hands into the floor behind the hips to help rotate the pelvis forward. If able to sit tall on the sitting bones with the hands off the floor, clasp and open the feet like a book, pressing the heels together while stretching the knees out toward the floor. Rotate the pelvis forward to draw the heart center toward the horizon.

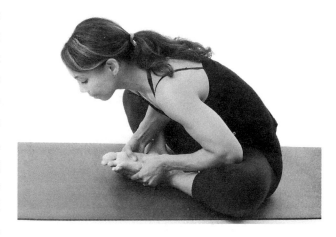

As a variation, invite students to play around with extending their arms fully forward, palms pressing down, using this alternative positioning to leverage the lifting of their heart center, elongation of their spine, and deeper forward rotation of their hips. Keeping the sitting bones rooted, heels pressing together, shoulder blades down the back, heart center open, move with the breath to lengthen the spine while folding forward from the hips. Use the elbows to press the thighs back, knees out, and chest forward. Create a feeling of bringing the belly button toward the toes, sternum to the horizon. Cueing this action will encourage students to minimize the rounding of their back and reduce potential strain in the lower back and neck. If students report pain in the inner knee or groin, encourage them to place blocks under their knees.

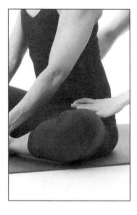

Use Hip Handles to cue the student's pelvis to neutrality.

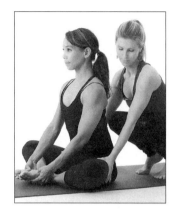

Apply Clasping Rotation to the student's upper thighs to assist their external rotation. Ask and re-ask the student about pressure in her knees and stop this adjustment if she reports tension in her knees.

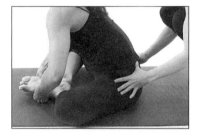

If your hands are large enough, apply an Opposite Rotation cue with your fingers cueing external rotation of the thighs and your thumbs sliding up the sacrum to cue anterior rotation of the pelvis.

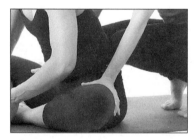

In Knees Up Stance, apply Clasping Rotation to the student's upper thighs while sliding your knees up from the upper back rim of the student's pelvis toward her lower back ribs (your knees just to the sides of the spine, not touching it at all).

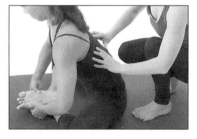

If the student is rounding her back, encourage her to rise up higher from the forward fold, using Finger Presses or Finger Draws to cue her shoulder blades down her back as she lifts her sternum.

Modification

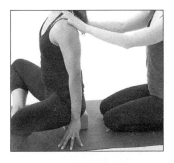

If the student is unable to sit up on the front of the sitting bones or if the knees are higher than the hips, offer a block or other bolster to place under the sitting bone, then use Hip Handles to guide the student to pelvic neutrality.

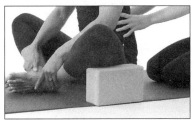

If the student reports issues or tension in the inner knees, offer blocks or other firm bolsters to place under the knees, then refocus on giving cues to highlight pelvic neutrality, a tall spine, and a spacious heart center.

Explore Further

Teaching Yoga: page 222

Yoga Sequencing: page 370

Teaching Yoga Resource Center:
   www.markstephensyoga.com/resources

Supta Baddha Konasana (Reclined Bound Angle Pose)

From the preparatory (upright) position for Baddha Konasana, verbally cue the student to recline back with the hands on the floor behind, then to release onto the elbows and then all the way to the floor. Provide props as indicated: blocks under the knees if there is intense pressure in the inner

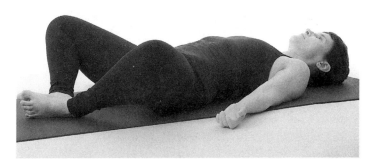

knees or thighs, and a bolster under the back and head if there is intense pressure in the lower back or neck.

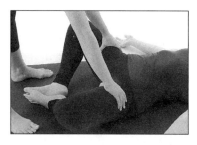

Place Light Hands on the student's thighs to encourage their external rotation and abduction while being sensitive to pressure in the knees.

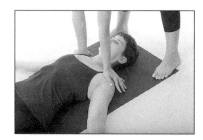

Use Light Hands to encourage the student to release the shoulders to the floor and allow the heart center to naturally expand.

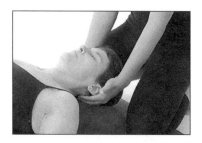

Place your fingertips up into the student's occipital ridge and lightly press while drawing more length to her neck.

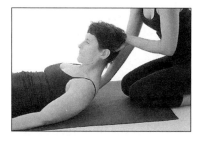

Use Light Hands under the student's back to help ease her back up to sitting.

Modification

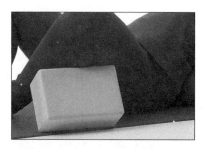

If the student reports issues or tension in the knees or inner thighs, offer blocks to place under the knees.

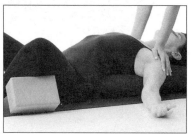

If the student is unable to recline onto the back free of tension in the knees and lower back, offer a bolster (or several) to place under the back.

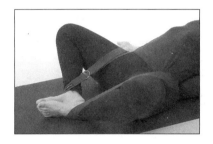

If the student releases back free of strain in the knees, offer a strap to place around the upper pelvis, over the thighs and ankles, and around and under the feet, cinching it to be taut before cueing to recline back.

Explore Further

Teaching Yoga: pages 326-29

Yoga Sequencing: page 428

Teaching Yoga Resource Center: www.markstephensyoga.com/resources

---

Ubhaya Padangusthasana (Both Big Toes Pose)

Sitting in Dandasana, verbally cue and demonstrate bending the knees to clasp the big toes with the middle and index fingers, then slowly extending the legs straight while pulling with the fingers to leverage the anterior rotation of the pelvis and the lifting and neutral extension of the spine. Then cue students to slowly bend the elbows and pull the sternum toward their toes.

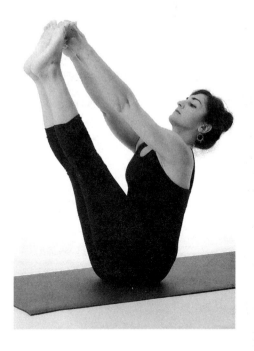

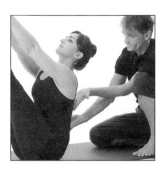

In the preparatory position, the student will clasp the big toes and extend the legs, spine, and arms. Most students tend to slump. Use a Light Hand to cue drawing the sacrum in (anterior rotation of the pelvis), while the other Light Hand slides up the thoracic spine to cue lifting the sternum.

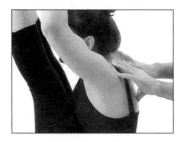

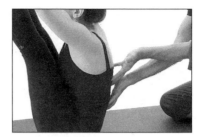

Verbally cueing the student to flex the elbows while drawing the sternum toward the toes, apply Light Hands to the tops of the shoulders to cue the shoulder down and away from the ears.

As the student draws the torso closer to the legs, the tendency is to slump. Again use a Light Hand on the sacrum but press more firmly and in an upward direction to counter the tendency to slump.

Modification

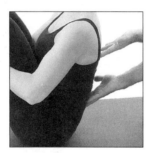

If the student in unable to clasp the big toes without bending the knees or slumping, verbally cue to bend the knees and clasp behind them while using a Light Hand on the sacrum to cue the anterior rotation of the pelvis.

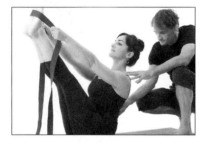

As a student with tight hamstrings progresses with the knee-clasping position, offer a strap around the feet and give the same tactile cue.

Explore Further

Yoga Sequencing: page 433

Teaching Yoga Resource Center:
www.markstephensyoga.com/resources

Urdhva Mukha Paschimottanasana
(Upward-Facing West Intense Stretch Pose)

Verbally cue and demonstrate preparing as for Ubhaya Padangusthasana, except rather than clasping the big toes, cue either clasping the sides of the feet or clasping one wrist around the feet. Then proceed as for Ubhaya Padangusthasana.

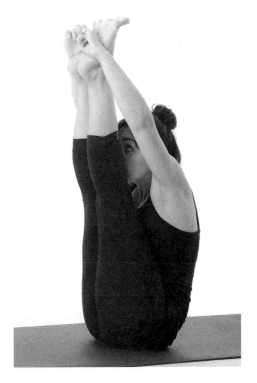

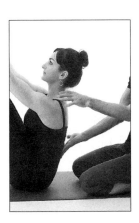

Use a Light Hand to cue drawing the sacrum in (anterior rotation of the pelvis) while the other Light Hand slides up the thoracic spine to cue lifting the sternum.

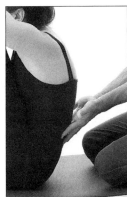

Verbally cueing the student to flex the elbows while drawing the sternum toward the toes, apply Light Hands to the tops of the shoulders to cue the shoulder down and away from the ears.

Modification

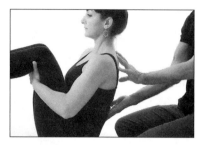

If the student is unable to clasp the fingers or wrist around the feet without bending the knees or slumping, verbally cue to bend the knees and clasp behind them while using a Light Hand on the sacrum to cue the anterior rotation of the pelvis.

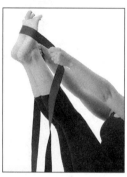

As a student with tight hamstrings progresses with the knee-clasping position, offer a strap around the feet and give the same tactile cue.

Explore Further

Yoga Sequencing: page 438

Teaching Yoga Resource Center:
www.markstephensyoga.com/resources

Supta Padangusthasana A and B (Reclined Big Toe Pose A and B)

Lying supine with the feet drawn in, as for Setu Bandha Sarvangasana (Bridge Pose), clasp the right foot and straighten the right leg (use a strap if needed). Move toward straightening the left leg onto the floor, pressing out through the heel while internally rotating the thigh and keeping the knee and toes pointing up. With an exhalation, bring the chin toward the shin while keep both legs straight and strong. Try to rotate the pubis forward and down while lifting the sternum away from the belly. Transition to the B variation by releasing the back to the floor, turning the head to the left and slowly extending the left leg out to the left in abduction. Be more interested in keeping the left buttock on the floor than getting the right leg farther over.

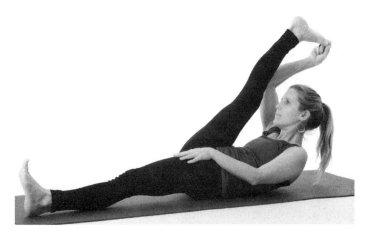

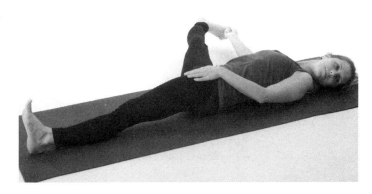

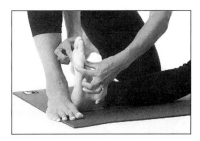

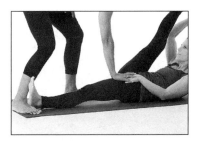

Place your foot against the student's left heel to encourage the student to press out through that heel, and use a Light Hand to orient the left toes and knee to point straight up, further cueing this alignment by lightly internally rotating that thigh.

As you verbally cue the student to lift the chin toward the shin on an exhalation (the A variation), keep pressing your foot against the heel and use Open Palms to press the left thigh down. Verbally encourage holding this position for five breaths before slowly releasing down in preparation for the B variation.

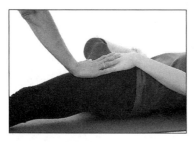

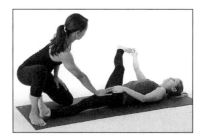

Verbally cue the student to feel the weight of the left buttock on the floor and to maintain with quality of grounding while extending the right leg to the right—only as far as the grounding of the left buttock doesn't change. Press an Open Palm on the student's thigh or hip to assist in maintaining this rooting action.

Verbally cue extending the right leg to the right and back up to the starting position five times before cueing the student to hold the leg out in the abducted position.

Modification

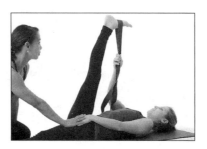

If the student is unable to clasp the right big toe and fully straighten that leg without the shoulder lifting off the floor, offer a strap to place around the foot and proceed with the same verbal and tactile cues.

Variation

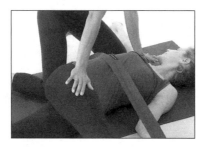

After holding the B variation for five breaths, draw the right leg up and across to the left, releasing the right arm over to the right onto the floor while using the left hand to draw the right leg across to the left, creating a simple twist that stretches the outside of the right leg.

Explore Further

Teaching Yoga: page 217

Yoga Sequencing: page 429

Teaching Yoga Resource Center:
www.markstephensyoga.com/resources

Apanasana (Wind-Relieving Pose or Knees to Chest Pose)

Lying on the back, draw the knees gently in toward the chest. Inhaling, release the knees slightly away from the chest; exhaling, hug them in. As simple as this appears, still counsel students to take it easy on the lower back. Play with rocking side to side or moving the knees around in circles to explore releasing tension in the lower back.

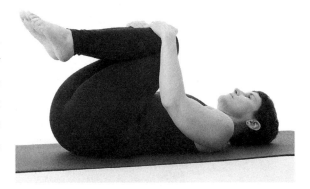

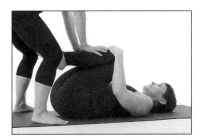

There is very little for the teacher to do with tactile cues with the student in this asana. Use very Light Hands to encourage drawing the thighs closer to the chest.

Explore Further

Teaching Yoga: page 216

Teaching Yoga Resource Center:
www.markstephensyoga.com/resources

Gomukhasana (Cow Face Pose)

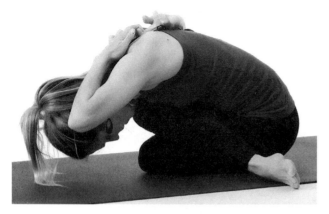

Prepare as for Ardha Matsyendrasana (Half Lord of the Fishes Pose), then draw the upper knee across the top of the lower knee with the heels close to the hips. If unable to fully cross the knees, come onto all fours to cross them; have a block waiting under the sitting bones before sitting back down. With the right knee on top, reach the left arm overhead, bending the elbow to draw the hand down the back while drawing the right arm back and reaching up to clasp the left fingers (use a strap if needed). Rooting the sitting bones, inhaling, lift the spine and chest; exhaling, fold forward. As with all seated forward bends, keep the sitting bones grounded while lengthening the spine and folding forward. Be sensitive to the knees, lower back, and shoulders. Keep the heart center open and the breath steady. Switch sides by either simply recrossing the legs, spinning 360 degrees, or pressing in Salamba Sirsasana II (Supported Headstand II) and recrossing the legs overhead.

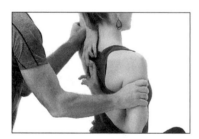

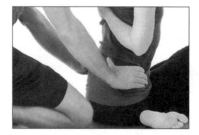

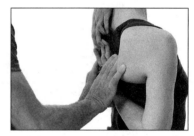

To assist the student with the arm positioning, use Clasping Rotation on the upper arms to assist their rotation, as follows: the lifted arm rotates externally, the other arm rotates internally.

Use Hip Handles with Clasping Rotation to cue the grounding and anterior rotation of the student's pelvis as the source of the forward fold.

If the student isn't ready to fold forward, apply Finger Draws on the shoulder blades to cue the shoulders down and away from the ears.

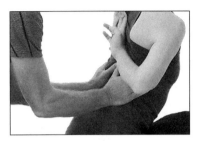

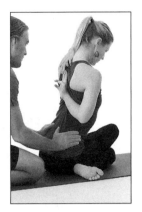

If the student can't fold forward, use Opposite Rotation along the side and back ribs to cue to lift the chest and lengthen the spine.

Reapply Hip Handles and reverse the Clasping Rotation to help ease the student back up to sitting.

Modification

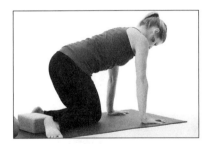

If the student is unable to sit tall on the sitting bones or is unable to cross the knees, cue to come forward onto the hands where the knees will far more easily cross over; offer this student a block between the heels so that the knees remain crossed while sitting back down and so the student doesn't slump in attempting to root the sitting bones.

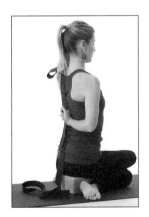

If the student is unable to clasp the fingers behind the back, offer a strap to extend between the hands.

Variation

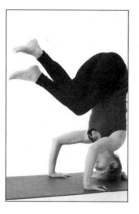

Transition to the other side through Sirsasana II (Headstand II).

Explore Further

Teaching Yoga: page 224

Yoga Sequencing: page 387

Teaching Yoga Resource Center: www.markstephensyoga.com/resources

---

Ardha Baddha Padma Paschimottanasana
(Half Bound Lotus West Intense Stretch Pose)

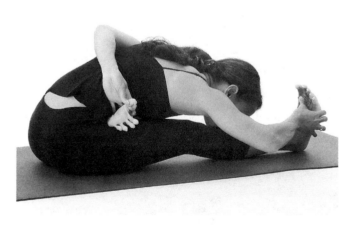

From Dandasana, instruct students to draw the right leg into half-lotus position, then to wrap the right arm behind the back to clasp the lotus foot. Rooting the sitting bones and keeping the extended leg active and internally rotating, inhaling, lift the spine and heart center; exhaling, fold forward. If the bent knee is off the floor, encourage the student to stay upright until the hip opens. Look for and cue a sense of symmetry amid the asymmetry of the asana.

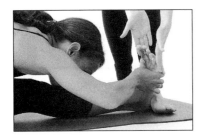

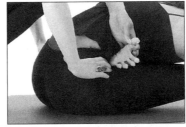

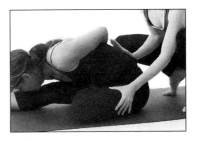

Place your foot against the student's left heel to encourage the student to press out through that heel, and use a Light Hand to orient the left toes and knee to point straight up, further cueing this alignment by lightly internally rotating that thigh.

Use Hip Handles to firmly root the sitting bones, and apply Clasping Rotation to encourage anterior rotation of the pelvis while verbally cueing the student to orient the sternum toward the left foot (not directly forward).

Use Clasping Rotation on the upper lotus thigh to support its external rotation while using a Finger Press on the student's lower back to encourage lifting up the lower back.

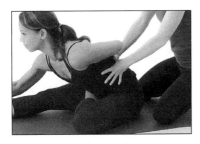

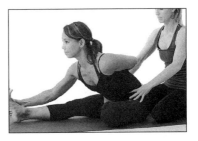

If the student can rotate the pelvis to bring the torso to forty-five degrees, verbally cue to begin folding through the spine with each exhalation, with the inhalation rising back toward the forty-five-degree angle to renew the lengthening of the spine and expansion of the heart center, continuing to move in this dynamic way with smaller and smaller movements. As the student inhales slightly up, apply an Opposite Rotation cue along the side ribs just below the apex of the curve in the spine to further convey the action of drawing the spine long even while folding forward.

Reapply Hip Handles with strong Clasping Rotation as you verbally cue the student to rise up from the forward fold on an inhalation, posteriorly rotating the pelvis to ease the transition up.

Modification

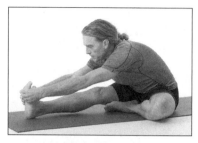

If unable to fold the legs into half lotus, guide the student to stay with Janu Sirsasana while continuing to open the internal rotators and adductors.

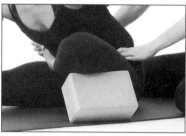

If the student's lotus knee is off the floor, offer a prop to place under it and do not press in any way that might increase pressure on that knee.

Explore Further

Teaching Yoga: page 225

Teaching Yoga Resource Center:
   www.markstephensyoga.com/resources

Agnistambhasana (Fire Log Pose or Two-Footed King Pigeon Pose)

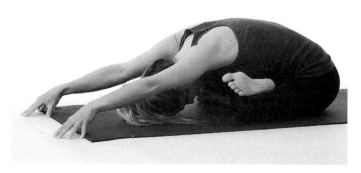

From a simple cross-legged position, place the hands on the floor behind the hips and lean back while sliding the heels forward to bring the shins parallel. Gradually rotate the pelvis forward to sit up taller. Once able to sit up with the hands free, stack the shins like logs with the ankles and knees atop each other on opposite sides. Fold forward. Keep the feet strongly flexed while engaging the muscles and ligaments around the knees, helping to protect the knees and accentuate the stretch in the hips.

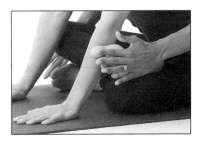

Use Light Hands to press the student's feet into full dorsiflexion while verbally cueing to maintain that action in the ankles.

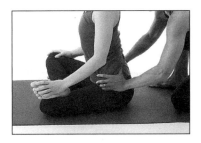

Verbally cue the student to root through the sitting bones while trying to rotate the pelvis forward, then use Hip Handles with Clasping Rotation to assist those actions while querying the student about any pressure or sharp pain in the knees (if there is any, back off).

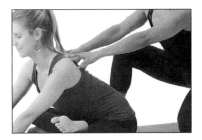

As the student rotates the pelvis forward, use Finger Draws or Light Hands to cue the shoulder blades down the back while verbally cueing to lift the sternum.

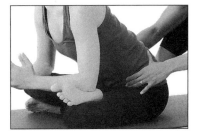

If the student is able to fold forward and place the elbows on the knees, verbally cue to press down onto the knees more firmly to leverage the sternum up as you reapply Hip Handles with Clasping Rotation to further encourage rotating the pelvis forward.

Modification

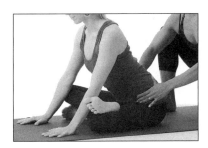

If the student is able to fold forward and place the hands on the floor in front of the legs, verbally cue to pull in on the fingertips to continue leveraging the sternum up while focusing the forward folding movement in the hip joints. Continue using Hip Handles with Clasping Rotation, reversing the actions in your hands to help ease the student back up.

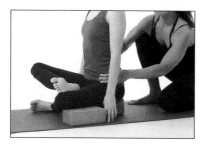

If the student is unable to cross the heels to the opposite knees, guide the student to stay with other cross-legged hip openers, especially Thread-the-Needle Pose. Also offer a block to place under the sitting bones if unable to sit up tall on the front of the sitting bones.

Explore Further

Teaching Yoga: page 227

Yoga Sequencing: page 362

Teaching Yoga Resource Center:
  www.markstephensyoga.com/resources

Eka Pada Raj Kapotasana I (One-Leg King Pigeon Pose I)

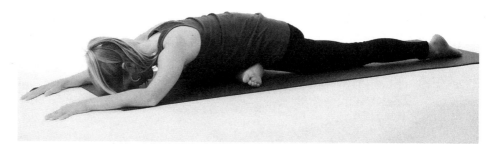

This hip opener is the preparatory position for the back bend of the same name, this being I rather than II. From Adho Mukha Svanasana (Downward-Facing Dog Pose), bring the right knee just outside the right hand while releasing the left hip and leg to the floor. Prop the left sitting bone as high as necessary to ensure that (a) the sitting bone is firmly supported, (b) the hips are even, and (c) there is no pressure on the inside of the right knee. Slowly fold forward and down.

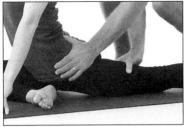

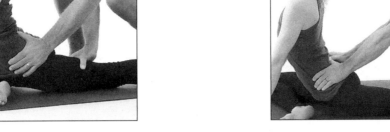

Use Light Hands to help position the student's extended leg straight back from the hip with the knee pointing straight down. Then verbally cue to root the foot down to leverage the internal rotation of that thigh, using Clasping Rotation on that thigh to assist this action.

Use Hip Handles to help position the student's hips level and even with each other, then press your thumbs down along the sacrum to create more space in the lower back.

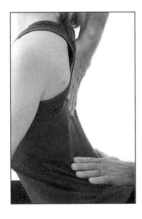

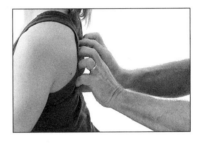

Use Finger Draws to cue the student's shoulder blades down the back.

Press an Open Palm on the student's sacrum with the pressure toward the heels while sliding the other Open Palm up the back, encouraging deeper release through the hips and up along the spine and torso.

Modification

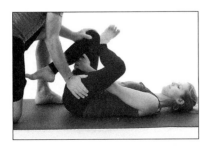

If the student reports tension in the front knee or if the hips are more than about six inches off the floor, encourage working with Sucirandhrasana until the hips open up more.

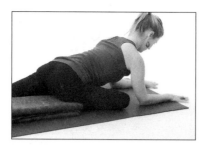

If the student is unable to ground the pelvis evenly to the floor, offer a block or blanket under the sitting bone of the bent leg to reduce pressure in that knee and in the sacroiliac joint.

Explore Further

Teaching Yoga: page 206
Yoga Sequencing: page 383
Teaching Yoga Resource Center:
www.markstephensyoga.com/resources

Eka Pada Sirsasana (One Leg behind Head Pose)

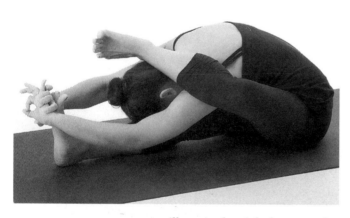

In Dandasana, slide the right foot in, clasping the knee to leverage the anterior rotation of the pelvis and extension of the spine. Do the first three preparatory steps described for Astavakrasana (Eight-Angle Pose) before drawing the lower right leg behind the right shoulder and across the back. Sit tall with the palms in anjali mudra before folding forward as described for Janu Sirsasana. Forcing this asana will strain the right knee, neck, and lower back. Keep the right foot strongly flexed to stabilize the knee. Use the lifting of the torso, elongation of the spine, and spreading of the collarbones to deepen the hip opening.

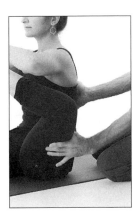

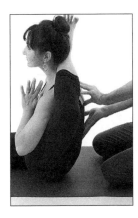

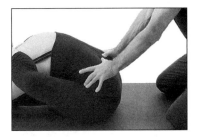

Assist with Light Hands in the student's effort to draw the leg behind the back. Use Clasping Rotation on that thigh to focus the effort in the external rotation of the hip, thereby reducing pressure in the knee. If the student's leg is touching the neck (rather than being against the back), encourage staying with hip openers before attempting this asana.

With the student's leg positioned behind the back, Apply Light Hands up from the lower back and down from the shoulders to encourage lifting tall through the spine and torso.

Use Hip Handles with Clasping Rotation to cue the anterior rotation of the student's pelvis as the source of the forward fold.

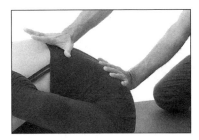

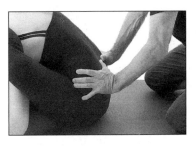

If the student folds farther than forty-five degrees forward, press an Open Palm on the sacrum with downward pressure while sliding the other Open Palm up the back from just below the apex of the curve in the back.

Reapply Hip Handles and reverse the Clasping Rotation to help ease the student back up to sitting.

Variation

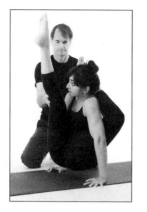

To offer an arm-support variation, cue drawing the torso back up, pressing the hands down, and straightening the arms to lift the hips off the floor, drawing the extended leg up to the chin into Chakorasana (Partridge Pose). From there, either transition to Chaturanga Dandasana to the asanas described below.

Explore Further

Teaching Yoga: pages 226-27

Yoga Sequencing: page 384

Teaching Yoga Resource Center: www.markstephensyoga.com/resources

---

Sukhasana (Simple Pose)

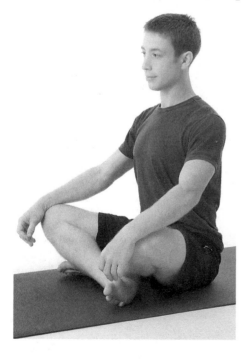

Sitting in Dandasana, verbally cue and demonstrate folding the legs into a simple cross-legged position.

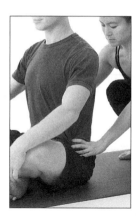

Use Hip Handles with Clasping Rotation to help root the student's sitting bones and to encourage the weight more to the front of the sitting bones.

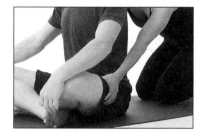

Apply Clasping Rotation to the student's upper thighs to assist their external rotation and abduction. Ask the student and ask again about pressure in the knees and stop this adjustment if the student reports tension in the knees.

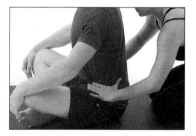

If your hands are large enough, apply an Opposite Rotation cue with your fingers, cueing external rotation of the thighs, and your thumbs sliding up the sacrum to cue anterior rotation of the pelvis to neutrality.

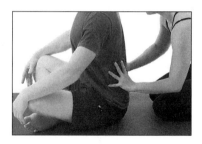

Use Finger Spreads between the upper rim of the student's pelvis to the lower rim of the ribs to cue lengthening up through the lower back.

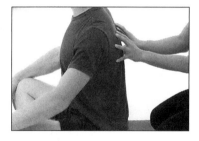

Use Finger Draws along the shoulder blades to cue the shoulder blades down against the back ribs while verbally cueing the student to lift through the core of the body without letting the lower front ribs protrude out.

Modification

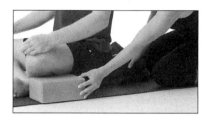

If the student reports tension in the inner knees or thighs, offer blocks under her knees.

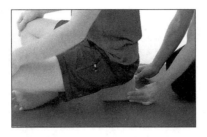

If the student is unable to sit on top of her sitting bones, offer her a block or other firm bolster to sit on.

Explore Further

Teaching Yoga Resource Center:
www.markstephensyoga.com/resources

Padmasana (Lotus Pose)

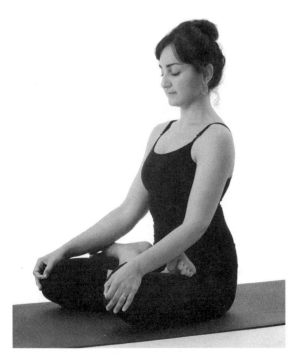

Teach Padmasana by cueing the release of the hips, never straining the knees. Ground the sitting bones and sit tall. From a simple cross-legged position, clasp the right heel and draw it toward the left hip. Relaxing in the right hip and inner thigh and groin, externally rotate the femur to release the right knee toward the floor. Proceed in the same way with the other leg. Ground through the sitting bones; keep cultivating pelvic neutrality, neutral spinal extension, and a spacious heart center. Never force the knees down. With the hands on the knees, cue gazing at the tip of the nose or to a point on the floor.

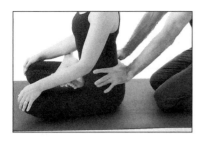

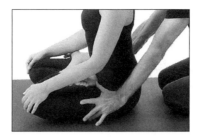

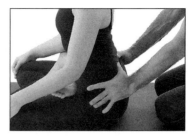

Use Hip Handles with Clasping Rotation to help root the student's sitting bones and to encourage the weight more to the front of the sitting bones.

Apply Clasping Rotation to the student's upper thighs to assist their external rotation. Ask the student and ask again about pressure in the knees and stop this adjustment if the student reports tension in the knees.

If your hands are large enough, apply an Opposite Rotation cue with your fingers cueing external rotation of the thighs and your thumbs sliding up the sacrum to cue anterior rotation of the pelvis.

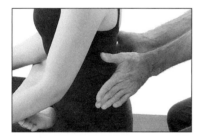

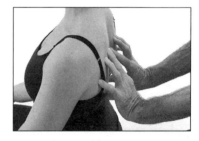

Use Hip Handles with Clasping Rotation to encourage maximum comfortable forward rotation of the pelvis as the primary source of the forward fold before placing the hands on the floor, blocks, or a wall.

While verbally cueing students, draw the spine long and sternum forward in the halfway-up position, using Opposite Rotation at the shoulder blades to cue the shoulder blades down the back and the sternum away from the belly, before cueing to fold farther down.

Modification

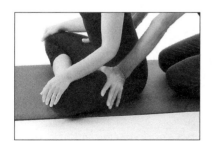

If the student is unable to fold the legs into full Lotus Pose, encourage exploring Ardha Padmasana (Half Lotus Pose) or Sukhasana.

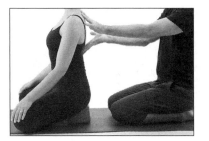

If the student is unable to sit on top of the sitting bones, offer a block or other firm bolster to sit on.

Explore Further

Teaching Yoga: page 225

Yoga Sequencing: page 404

Teaching Yoga Resource Center:
www.markstephensyoga.com/resources

Baddha Padmasana (Bound Lotus Pose)

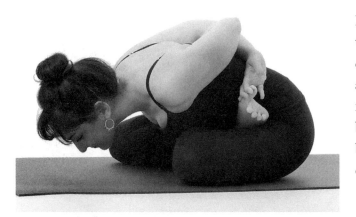

From Padmasana, reach the arms behind the back to clasp the feet. If unable to clasp the feet, clasp the elbows or forearms. Inhaling, extend the spine; exhaling, fold forward. Try to stay for ten slow breaths, using this asana to refine the breath and move into a deeper and quieter space inside.

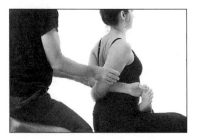

Use Clasping Rotation on the student's upper arms to assist their internal rotation as the student brings the arms around the back.

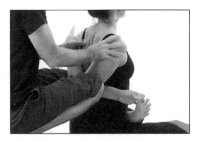

Use Hip Handles with Clasping Rotation to cue the grounding and anterior rotation of the student's pelvis as the source of the forward fold.

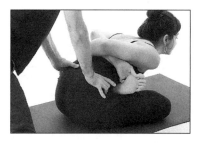

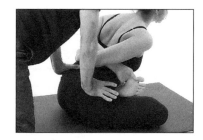

Use Hip Handles with Clasping Rotation to cue the grounding and anterior rotation of the student's pelvis as the source of the forward fold.

Reapply Hip Handles and reverse the Clasping Rotation to help ease the student back up to sitting.

Modification

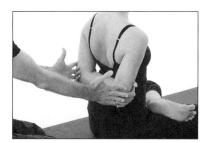

If the student is unable to wrap the arms around the back to clasp the feet, either offer a strap around the feet or cue to clasp the elbows.

Variation

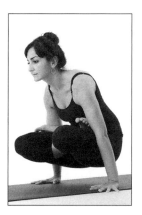

After drawing back up to sitting upright, release the hands to the floor by the hips and press firmly through the hands lift into Tolasana (Scales Pose) for 108 rounds of kapalabhati pranayama.

Explore Further

Teaching Yoga: page 226

Teaching Yoga Resource Center:
   www.markstephensyoga.com/resources

Hanumanasana (Divine Monkey Pose)

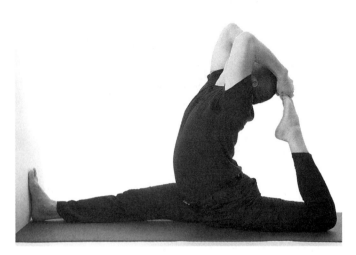

From Anjaneyasana, place the hands on the floor and shift the hips back above the rear knee while straightening the front leg. Stay here for one to two minutes. Keeping the hips even with the front of the mat, slowly slide the heel of the front leg forward while extending the rear leg. Since most students are unable to release fully into this asana, offer blocks to place (1) under the sitting bone of the front leg and/or (2) on both sides of the hips for hand support. It is important to position the hips even with the front of the mat while the sitting bone of the front leg is firmly grounded, thereby creating a symmetrical foundation for spinal extension and reducing the risk of lower-back strain. Once stably positioned with the spine upright, increasingly flex the front foot, engaging the quadriceps muscles and releasing the hamstrings. To the extent that the hips are even with the front of the mat, the back leg will more easily extend straight back from the hip. Emphasize internal rotation of the back leg, especially if exploring the back-bend variation.

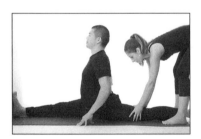 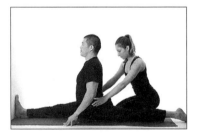 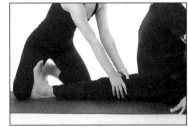

Use Light Hands to help position the student's back leg straight back from the hip with the knee pointing straight down. Then verbally cue the student to root the foot down to leverage the internal rotation of that thigh, using Clasping Rotation on that thigh to assist this action.

Use Hip Handles to help position the student's hips level and even with each other, then press your thumbs down along the sacrum to create more space in the lower back and cue movement toward pelvis neutrality.

Placing your knee or foot against the heel of the student's front leg, verbally cue pressing out through that heel and internally rotating that thigh, assisting this with Clasping Rotation on that thigh.

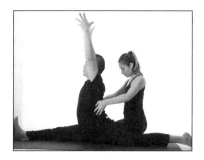

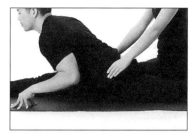

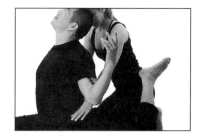

Sitting in Noose Stance and thereby positioning yourself in closer behind the student, use Finger Spreads between the pelvis and the side ribs to cue lifting through the spine and torso.

For the forward-fold expression of this asana, use Hip Handles to cue movement from the pelvis while keeping the pelvis level and even (the side of the back leg will tend to shift back).

For the back-bend expression of this asana, steady the student's balance with Hip Handles before guiding the hands to the lifted foot.

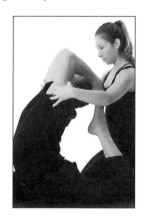

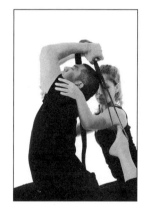

In the back bend, use Clasping Rotation on the upper arms to assist their external rotation and to help draw the student's elbows together as he or she eases the head back toward the foot.

Use Hip Handles to help stabilize the student's lateral balance as he or she slowly releases from the back bend.

Modification

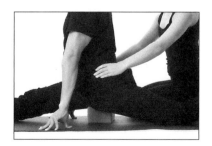

Offer blocks under the sitting bone of the front leg if the student is unable to ground that sitting bone to the floor with a level and even pelvis.

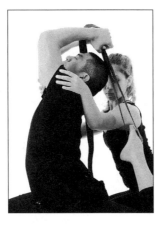

Offer a strap around the lifted foot for the student to clasp with both hands overhead if the student is unable to clasp the foot with both hands.

Explore Further

Teaching Yoga: page 221

Yoga Sequencing: page 389

Teaching Yoga Resource Center:
   www.markstephensyoga.com/resources

Chapter 10

Inversions

When we go upside down, the world appears to be inverted. Here even the simplest of movements can be confusing as we experience this opposite and unfamiliar relationship to gravity. This shift in perspective and neuromuscular awareness creates an opportunity to further expand our sense of being in the world while reversing the effects of gravity in the body. The brain is flushed with nourishing blood, the mind clears, the nerves quiet down, and everything seems to become more still yet awake, offering a graceful invitation to meditation. With practice, even what is at first the most challenging inversion—Salamba Sirsasana (Supported Headstand)—becomes as stable its opposite, Tadasana (Mountain Pose), allowing students to remain in this asana for several minutes at a time. Whether in Sirsasana or Salamba Sarvangasana (Supported Shoulder Stand), students develop more nuanced muscular coordination that adds stability and ease to a variety of other asanas, including in fluid movements into and out of Adho Mukha Vrksasana (Handstand).

The greatest physical risk in inversions is to the neck (this does not apply to Viparita Karani, Active Reversal Pose). It is very important to give students clear and methodical guidance in setting up for inversions in a way that minimizes this risk. Students with cervical spine issues are advised not to practice any asanas that further strain the neck.

Inversion and Menstruation

There is considerable confusion and disagreement among yoga teachers over whether women should practice full inversions when menstruating. Some assert that inversions reverse the flow of menses, often going further by maintaining that this retrograde menstruation can cause endometriosis. However, there is no medical evidence showing that inversion disrupts the natural flow of menses. If there were such evidence, then even Adho Mukha Svanasana (Downward-Facing Dog Pose) would be contraindicated when menstruating, and one would have to question even the effects of lying on the belly versus the back since the uterus and vagina are turned in opposite relationship to gravity.

Looking further into the question of menstruation in relationship to gravity, the NASA Medical Division has found no changes in menstrual flow among women in zero-gravity environments, pointing to intravaginal peristaltic muscular contraction and internal pressure, not a relationship to gravity, as the cause of normal menstrual egress. This is also why four-legged mammals have no problem with healthy menstrual flow despite not having a vertical orientation to gravity, and why a menstruating woman will flow just as normally whether sleeping on her back or on her belly despite her uterus and vagina being turned in opposite relation to gravity.

In advising students on the question of menstruation and inversion, veteran yoga teacher Barbara Benagh (2003) says that since "no studies or research make a compelling argument to avoid inversions during menstruation, and since menstruation affects each woman differently and can vary from cycle to cycle, I am of the opinion that each woman is responsible for her own decision."

Students who are not practicing Sirsasana or Salamba Sarvangasana can receive most of the benefits of full inversion in Viparita Karani (Active Reversal Pose, "the action or doing of reversing, turning upside down"), perhaps the most calming and deeply restorative asana, included below along with the other inversions. This is an excellent asana for all students, especially following a vigorous practice, stressful day, or when feeling energetically down.

Halasana (Plow Pose)

Lying supine, press the palms down, and with an exhalation, bring the feet overhead to the floor (or to a block, chair, or wall). Interlace the fingers behind the back and slightly shrug the shoulders under to draw weight more onto the shoulders. If there is pressure on the neck or upper spine, either release from this position or reset with one or two folded blankets placed under the arms and shoulders.

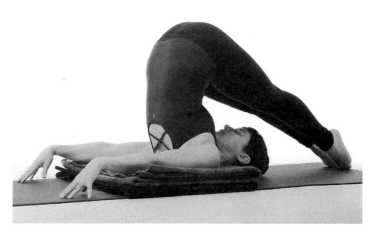

Press the feet firmly down (if possible, pointed back) to engage and press the thighs up, drawing the pubic bone away from the belly in lengthening the spine. Keep the arms and feet firmly grounding. Draw the collarbones down while spreading across the chest and pressing the spine through toward the heart. Keep pressing the sitting bones up, lengthening through the spine.

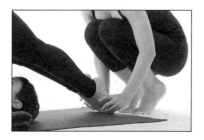

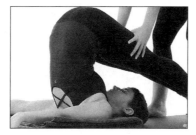

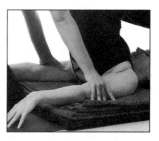

Use Light Hands to cue pressing down through the feet to leverage the full extension and awakening of the legs, verbally cueing the student to press the pubic bone away from the belly and thus draw more length into the lower back as the sitting bones rise farther over the shoulders.

Apply Clasping Rotation to the student's thighs to cue their internal rotation, which will make the further anterior rotation of the pelvis toward neutrality more accessible.

Press Light Hands onto the student's arms to encourage their active grounding.

Explore Further

Teaching Yoga: page 231
Yoga Sequencing: page 388
Teaching Yoga Resource Center:
  www.markstephensyoga.com/resources

Salamba Sarvangasana (Supported Shoulder Stand)

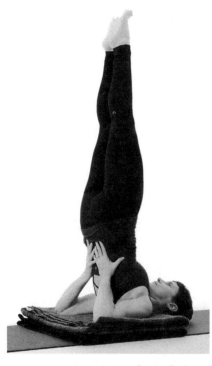

In practicing Salamba Sarvangasana, most students' necks will press into the floor. Over time, with openness and strength in the upper back, shoulders, arms, and chest, their neck will not press into the floor. Until that develops, or if there is any discomfort in the neck, instruct students to set up a platform using folded blankets, then lie down with their shoulders in about three inches from the edge of the blankets. Once their legs are brought overhead, their shoulders should remain on the platform, the neck free, and the head on the floor. From there, instruct as follows:

With the arms down by the sides, on an exhalation press into the palms and slowly draw the legs overhead into Halasana. If the feet do not reach the floor, either support the hips with the hands and elbows in Ardha Sarvangasana (Half Shoulder Stand), or come down and practice with a chair or the wall overhead for the feet. With the feet on the floor overhead, interlace the fingers behind the back and slightly shrug the shoulders under to bring the weight of the body more onto the shoulders and off the neck. Press the feet firmly down into the floor to activate the legs, pressing the tops of the femurs up to help rotate the pelvis anteriorly and thereby draw more length through the lumbar spine. If possible, do this with the feet pointed in plantar flexion; if necessary, keep the toes curled under and consider placing them on a block, chair, or wall.

Now place the hands on the back as close to the floor as possible, supporting the back, and slowly extend the legs up toward the sky (the easiest method is with the knees bent and using one leg at a time, then over time with straight legs moving up together).

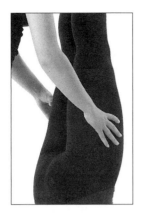

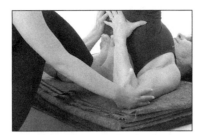

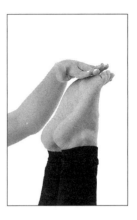

Use Clasping Rotation on the student's thighs to cue the legs together and to cue their slight internal rotation.

Sitting on the floor behind the student's back, place your feet on the back below where the student has placed the hands and clasp the elbows. As you slowly slide your feet up the back (to the sides of the spine, not against it), use your hands to bring the elbows into or toward alignment with the shoulders.

While first verbally cueing the student to dorsiflex the ankles, use Light Hands on the heels along with a verbal cue to press out through the heels, then use Finger Flicks to cue spreading the toes while verbally cueing to press out more through the balls of the feet.

Modification

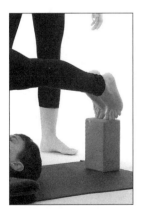

If a student is unable to bring the feet overhead to the floor into Halasana, invite the student to explore near a wall where he or she can place the feet on the wall (or offer a chair, block, or other firm prop to place under the feet).

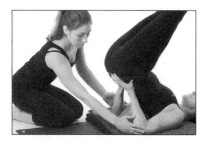

If a student is unable to bring the feet overhead to the floor into Halasana and is not using a wall, chair, of block to prop the feet, cue to place the hands under the hips and come into a jack-knife position (Ardha Sarvangasana).

Explore Further

Teaching Yoga: page 232

Yoga Sequencing: page 422

Teaching Yoga Resource Center:
www.markstephensyoga.com/resources

Karnapidasana (Ear-Squeezing Pose)

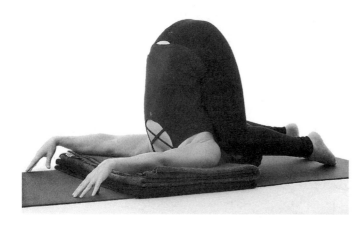

From Halasana, cue students to release the knees toward or to the ears while pressing the arms down into the floor, and to squeeze the knees into the ears while listening to the breath from inside. Encourage keeping the breath full and being very sensitive to undue pressure in the neck or lower back.

Rather than offering any tactile cues, focus on the general verbal cues for this asana.

Explore Further

Teaching Yoga: page 232

Yoga Sequencing: page 392

Teaching Yoga Resource Center:
www.markstephensyoga.com/resources

Urdhva Padmasana (Upward Lotus Pose)

Exploring from Salamba Sarvangasana (Shoulder Stand), draw the legs into Padmasana (Lotus Pose) position, using one hand at a time to assist if necessary. Stretch the lotus knees straight up, then extend an arm straight up and bring the knee on that side to the hand, then place the other hand and knee together. Focus on rooting the shoulders, expanding the chest, extending the spine, and holding steady while breathing smoothly and spaciously. Engage mula bandha and gaze to the nose or belly.

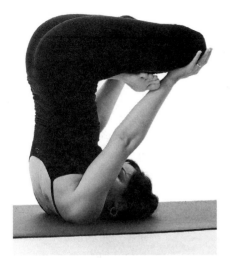

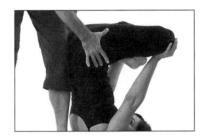

As students first explore this asana, stand with the side of your leg against their back and use Hip Handles to assist them in finding balance on their shoulders and head. Keeping your leg against the student's back, as light as possible as they come more into their controlled balance, use Light Hands along the student's thighs (close to her knees) to help her position her hands more squarely under her knees.

Variation

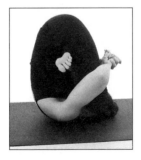

Explore folding more deeply into Pindasana (Embryo Pose).

Explore Further

Teaching Yoga: page 232

Yoga Sequencing: page 440

Teaching Yoga Resource Center: www.markstephensyoga.com/resources

---

Salamba Sirsasana I (Supported Headstand I)

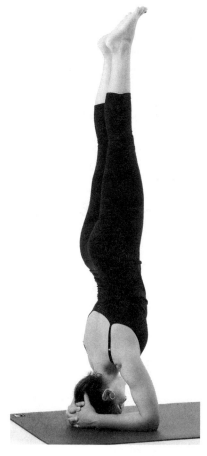

If students are new to Salamba Sirsasana I, have them practice next to a wall. Instruct two basic roots: the forearms and crown of the head, starting with the positioning of the arms with the elbows shoulder distance apart. Begin with the knees and forearms on the floor. In interlacing the fingers, instruct students to keep the palms wide open and their fingers sufficiently loose to be able to firmly root down from the ulnar side of the wrists to the elbows. The top of the head should be placed directly down on the floor with the back of the head braced lightly by the base of the thumbs. Ask students to slowly straighten their legs while pressing firmly down through their forearms and drawing their shoulder blades down against their back ribs, their shoulders drawing away from their wrists. Maintaining this position, guide students to walk their feet in toward their elbows until bringing their hips as high as possible over their shoulders; encourage students to keep the spine long in this transition. Encourage steady ujjayi pranayama and *dristana*. Rooting down more firmly through the elbows, ask students to try to draw their knees in toward the chest and the heels toward the hips, and then to rotate the pelvis up and slowly extend the legs straight up toward the sky. Once upside down, bring awareness back to the roots in the forearms, and cue students to create a feeling of pulling the elbows toward each other without actually moving them; this will broaden the shoulders, activate the latissimus dorsi muscles, and add stability.

Now accentuate the other source of rooting: press the top of the head fairly firmly down, thereby triggering the roots-and-extension effect, activating the spinal erector and multifidus muscles close to the spine. This will relieve pressure in the neck, elongate the entire spine, and create a feeling of grounded levity. Finally, instruct students to bring their ankles together, strongly flex their feet (toes toward the shins), and energetically extend out through their heels before pointing the feet and spreading the toes like lotus petals. In releasing from Salamba Sirsasana I, the easiest method is to bend the knees and draw them toward the chest, slowly lowering into Balasana (Child's Pose).

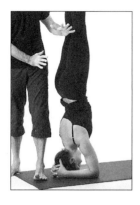

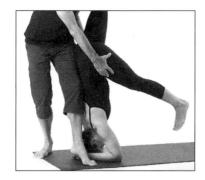

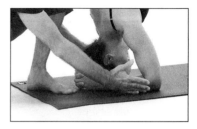

In working with students who are new to exploring Salamba Sirsasana away from the wall, simply stand behind them to ensure they do not fall over backward.

To assist a student in coming up into Salamba Sirsasana, stand behind and turn sideways so you can press the side of your leg or knee against the back as a source of stability, then as the student walks the feet toward the hands, give further assistance to balance while using your hands to assist in drawing the legs overhead.

Use Light Hands to cue the energetic action of drawing the elbows as though toward each other (without them actually moving).

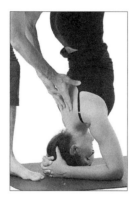

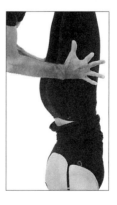

Use Finger Draws below the student's neck to cue drawing the shoulders away from the wrists and thereby create more space around the neck.

Use Clasping Rotation at the student's hips to position the pelvis neutrally in relation to the spine.

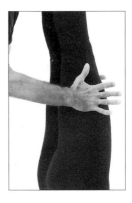

Use Open Palms along the student's legs to cue them into alignment.

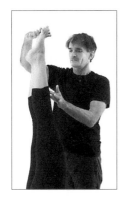

While first verbally cueing the student to dorsiflex the ankles, use Light Hands on the heels along with a verbal cue to press out through the heels, then use Finger Flicks to cue spreading the toes while verbally cueing to press out more through the balls of the feet.

Explore Further

Teaching Yoga: page 233
Yoga Sequencing: page 422
Teaching Yoga Resource Center: www.markstephensyoga.com/resources

---

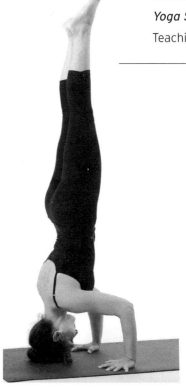

Salamba Sirsasana II (Supported Headstand II)

From all fours, cue placing the top of the head and the hands on the floor with the head and the wrists forming the points of a triangle. Keep the wrists under the elbows and in line with the shoulders while drawing the shoulder blades firmly down against the back ribs. Curl the toes under, straighten the legs, and slowly bring the feet toward the elbows to elevate the hips over the shoulders. Pressing firmly down through the head and hands, extend the legs overhead. As in Salamba Sirsasana I, root the top of the head to elongate the spine. Keep the elbows from splaying out while keeping the shoulder blades firmly against the back ribs. Activate the legs as in Salamba Sirsasana I. With stability and ease, explore using this asana as the base for exploring a variety of arm balances.

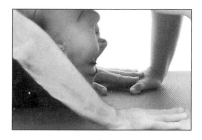

Press Light Hands onto the student's hands to cue their equal rooting.

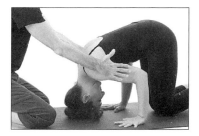

Press Light Hands against the student's elbows to cue them into alignment with the shoulders.

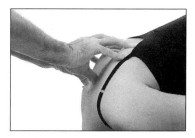

Use Finger Draws on the student's shoulder blades to cue them down against the back ribs, thereby reducing pressure on the neck.

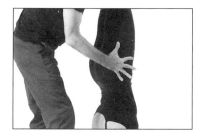

Use Clasping Rotation at the student's hips to position the pelvis neutrally in relation to the spine.

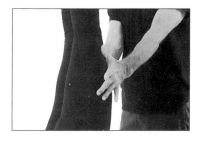

Use Open Palms along the student's legs to cue them into alignment.

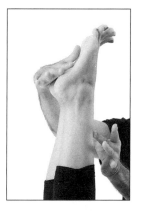

While first verbally cueing the student to dorsiflex the ankles, use Light Hands on the heels along with a verbal cue to press out through the heels, then use Finger Flicks to cue spreading the toes while verbally cueing to press out more through the balls of the feet.

Explore Further

Teaching Yoga: page 234

Yoga Sequencing: page 423

Teaching Yoga Resource Center:
    www.markstephensyoga.com/resources

Viparita Karani (Active Reversal Pose)

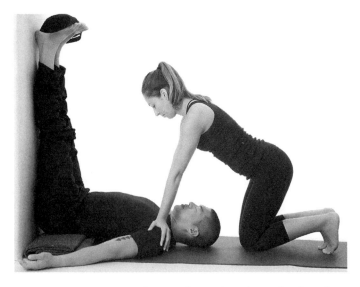

Sitting sideways next to a wall, slowly recline onto the back while swiveling the hips toward the wall and extending the legs up the wall. If tight hamstrings do not allow the legs to extend up with the buttocks touching the wall, slide the hips out away from the wall. Place a folded blanket under the lower back to create more ease through the lower back and sacrum. The palms can rest on the belly and heart, or drape the arms onto the floor, palms turned up. The legs can be held together with a strap and a sandbag placed on the feet for stability. Play with positioning the legs as for Baddha Konasana (Bound Angle Pose) or Upavista Konasana (Wide-Angle Forward Fold Pose).

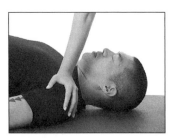

Press Light Hands onto the student's shoulders to cue letting go across the collarbones and relaxing across the chest.

Modification

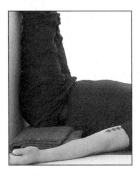

If the student in unable to position the hips against the wall with the legs straight up the wall, elevate the pelvis on a bolster and explore having the hips out several inches or more from the wall.

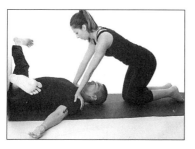

Offer the Upavista Konasana positioning of the legs.

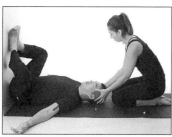

Offer the Baddha Konasana positioning of the legs.

Explore Further

Teaching Yoga: page 231
Yoga Sequencing: page 450
Teaching Yoga Resource Center:
  www.markstephensyoga.com/resources

Savasana (Corpse Pose or Final Relaxation Pose)

Savasana (from *sava*, "corpse") is the ultimate asana for reintegration after practicing other asanas and pranayama. Ask students to lie onto their backs and spread out as comfortably as possible with their arms draped onto the floor and palms facing up. If they feel any discomfort in the lower back, suggest placing a rolled blanket under their knees. Lift the chest a little to let the shoulder

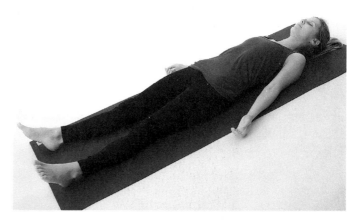

blades relax slightly toward each other, then lie back down with more spaciousness across the heart center. Take one last deep inhale, then with the exhalation, let everything go, starting with allowing the breath to flow however it naturally will. Give minimal guidance in cueing students to scan and release tension all through their bodies. There is finally no need for the muscles to do anything at all. Encourage students simply to watch what is happening. Suggest a sense of all the muscles and bones letting go of each other, a sense of detachment all through the body. Similarly, as naturally as thoughts come and go, encourage letting the thoughts flow, interested without being attached, becoming stiller, quieter, and clearer—breath by effortless breath. Stay in Savasana for at least five minutes. If students must leave class early, encourage them to rest in Savasana before leaving.

Gently awaken the class from Savasana with a soft voice, bringing awareness back to the breath. Suggest feeling the simple rising and falling of the chest and belly, cueing the class to gradually breathe more deeply and consciously, using the breath to reawaken awareness in the bodymind while changing as little as possible. Suggest bringing small movements into the fingers, hands, toes, and feet. With a deep inhalation, suggest stretching the arms overhead before rolling onto the right side, curling up, and nurturing oneself for a few breaths before slowly coming up to sitting. Now is an ideal time to meditate.

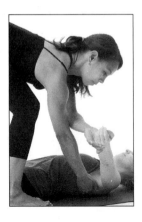

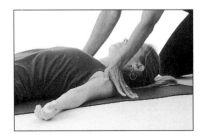

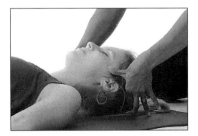

Lift the student's arm and slide a Light Hand down along that shoulder blade while lightly placing the student's arm back onto the floor, then do the same on the other side, creating more space across the heart center.

With Light Hands on the student's shoulders, press the shoulders lightly down.

Slide your thumbs across the student's temples, and /or press your thumb tip onto the third eye for a few seconds before lightly letting go.

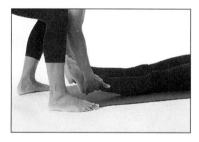

Gently lift the student's legs, move them slowly side-to-side, then place them lightly back onto the floor however wide apart the student initially had them placed.

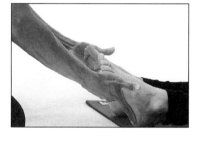

Squeeze the feet, and then let them go.

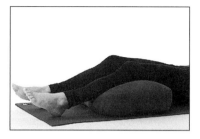

If the student feels any discomfort in the lower back or has lower-back issues, offer a bolster to place across under the knees.

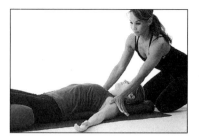

If the student wants a more heart- and breath-opening Savasana, suggest placing a low bolster or folded blanket along under the spine or across under the shoulder blades.

Explore Further

Teaching Yoga: page 234

Yoga Sequencing: pages 88-89, 425

Teaching Yoga Resource Center:
  www.markstephensyoga.com/resources

Part III
Evolution

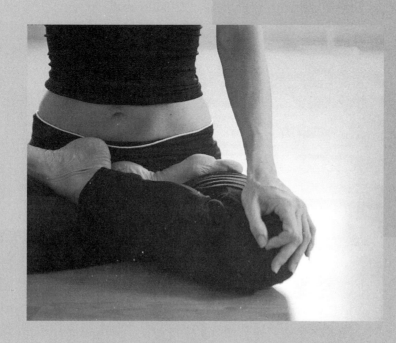

Chapter 11

Guiding Yoga in the Twenty-First Century

EARLY IN THIS BOOK I NOTED THAT YOGA HAS EVOLVED more in the last seventy-five years than in the previous thousand years. This assertion deserves some explanation in order to shed light on what this might mean for teachers and teaching in the present day and going forward. What are the evolutionary trends? How is yoga changing? As yoga teachers, what might we anticipate in the coming years, and where are we in the evolutionary process of yoga?

In nearly every field of human endeavor, we find various perspectives that attempt to define or at least characterize what it is all about, including where it came from and where it is headed. With respect to yoga, there is a tremendous diversity of views about how and where it originated and how it has evolved. Much of the literature and commentary on the origins and historical development of yoga rest on assertion or conjecture rather than careful research and methodical consideration of the evidence. This tendency has generated many fascinating stories about the history of yoga practice and teaching, many of which contain beautiful and inspirational myths that for many people are at the heart of their sense of it all. Even suggesting the questions posed here can be anathema to all that yoga means to some people, even irreverent given the religious tenacity with which some cling to their beliefs about yoga.

While respecting even the most mythical or fundamentalist of yoga beliefs, we can now confidently state that one of the most common and enduring yoga myths is that there is one yoga, or that some idealized, unadulterated form of yoga has evolved in a unilineal or unilinear fashion going back thousands of years. The romantic notion that there is "one yoga" that has evolved in such a way is explored in yoga scholar David Gordon White's recent anthology *Yoga in Practice* (2012). Noting that "people have 'reinvented' yoga in their own image" for at least two thousand years and that "every group in every age has created its own version and its own vision of yoga," White and the contributors to his anthology dig into the historical sources to reveal a diverse array of practices that are just as likely to have missed one another like the proverbial ships in the night than to have cross-fertilized, all evolving in ways punctuated or even defined more by discontinuity than with a consistent thread of technique or even purpose.

Appreciated in this way, yoga is a richly textured mosaic of practices that may or may not overlay, inform, or otherwise relate to one another. Still, White (2012, 6–11) suggests that we can distill four principles that have "persisted through time and across traditions":

1. Yoga as an analysis of perfection and cognition
2. Yoga as the raising and expansion of consciousness
3. Yoga as a path to omniscience
4. Yoga as a technique for supernatural accomplishment

Since here we are mostly interested in Hatha yoga and in particular its postural practices, for now we can consider the evolution of asana practices, which White and others, including Singleton (2010), show are first described only in the first millennium CE, not thousands of years earlier.[1] Yet in the contemporary literature of yoga we are often told that "the practice"—what we are doing today in yoga classes all around the world—is essentially the same as the yoga practiced thousands of years ago.[2] Such assertions are typically tied to claims of true or correct practice—what Singleton terms "orthopraxy"—that various styles and lineages assert in order to claim greater legitimacy, especially when the assertion includes direct transmission of the practice through a lineage, gurus, or a divine source. If my style of yoga is three thousand years old and yours is only thirty years old, then mine is purer since it is somehow more connected to an original form of yoga as it first manifested in the world.

These are not merely academic questions (although, to the extent that they are, they are increasingly informed by research that meets high standards of scholarship). Rather, these are profoundly practical questions that can very much affect how one comes to the practice and how one shares the practice with others. Approaches to yoga that claim they are somehow original, true, or correct are typically committed to preserving the practice in its idealized (if mythologized) form by transmitting it in specific and often strict ways from guru to disciple—terms that are heavily weighted with meaning and power. This is an especially practical matter as it so powerfully determines how students come to experience their yoga practice.

In its noun form, the Sanskrit term *guru* means "one who shares knowledge," while as an adjective it means "heavy" or "weighty" in reference to spiritual knowledge.[3] Some have suggested that the separate syllables *gu* and *ru* refer to dark and light, with the role of the guru being to impart the light of transcendental knowledge (Grimes 1996, 133). Regardless of etymology or specific definition, the relationship between guru and disciple is commonly one of the guru as the disciple's ultimate source of learning or awakening, which is said to be viable only if the guru is genuine and the disciple obedient and devoted to the guru's teachings. Rather than questioning the guru's understandings or methods, the disciple must only absorb them in practice.

One might find a sense of spiritual, paternal, or maternal comfort in the care of a guru or other spiritual guide who provides answers to all of the most basic or deepest questions of daily life. In explaining the benefits she has found in following a guru, a follower of Paramahansa Yogananda states that in having a guru, you "stop seeking and searching various paths and you have this one goal that you can wholeheartedly follow, trusting your guru to take you to the final goal of Yoga."[4] Surely there are many people for whom this resonates, particularly those who feel the need for a certain path along which any difficulties can be clearly explained through an appeal to the beliefs or liturgy of the guru. Surrendering completely to the wisdom and authority of the guru, believing wholly in the guru's teachings and thus feeling more fully the claimed truth of the one path, one might find liberation from routine distractions that allows a sense of purity in one's practice. Surrendering to a guru can also be problematic, especially if the guru abuses his or her power, which some observers have cogently argued is a common tendency in the guru-disciple relationship.[5]

There are other paths. As discussed above, there are not only many paths, but it is very likely that all paths are continuously evolving, even if there is much effort made to preserve what one believes to be a pure or correct path. As we arrived in the twentieth century, yoga was just coming to the West, where soon it would diversify and multiply in ways likely unimaginable even to those for whom practicing yoga was then a radical departure from the known diverse cultures of physical and spiritual practice. Much to the dismay of those holding fast to fundamentalist yoga beliefs, the attitude of open-minded experimentation with yoga practices was on wide display by the 1920s. Nearly a century later, this experimentation is contributing to the greatest creative evolution of yoga practice in the history of yoga.

Why? While the reality of yoga history is that yoga has always evolved through the creative explorations and new experiences of those deeply into the practice, today there are tens of millions of people worldwide stepping onto yoga mats with some intention related to living a better life. On every continent, in nearly every culture, across the cycles of life and the patterns of gender, ethnicity, religion, and belief, we find people practicing yoga. In practicing yoga, people are making choices about their practice that are related to the other realities of their lives: where they are, their values, their immediate needs and goals. In the spirit of human endeavor to have greater clarity, meaning, and well-being in life, we find that people modify what they are learning from their teachers, books, and other sources. In some instances the modifications are designed to make the practice more accessible, as in the pioneering creativity of Tiramulai Krishnamacharya (who created Ashtanga Vinyasa as an original synthesis of various forms of physical culture) or that of his student, B. K. S. Iyengar, who has given us most of the world of yoga props. In many instances we find innovations that tap into the wells of insight found in other practices, including dance, acrobatics, gymnastics, and the martial arts, various religious rituals and observances, and forms that can make it difficult to discern any element of yoga.[6]

Whenever someone shows up in the practice, he or she is at least potentially contributing to the creative evolution of yoga practice. As teachers—in contrast to gurus—we might well best open ourselves to working with our students in a way that supports them in the ways they are evolving their own practice, even as we contribute to this expansive evolution through the ways we create class sequences, provide narrative overlays to those sequences, share insights, and bring in qualities that derive from multiple varied sources found in the world's richly diverse cultures and in our own creative imaginations. While many on the fundamentalist paths will likely denounce such creativity as sacrilegious, it is likely that yoga will continue to evolve in myriad ways.

With more and more students opting for open-minded teachers on a consciously evolving path rather than gurus claiming to transmit pure ancient teachings, students are increasingly setting higher standards for teachers' overall knowledge and technical skill. An important facet of contemporary yoga evolution shines forth from the rapidly expanding fields of insight into the nature and functioning of the bodymind that is abundantly available for teachers to learn. With this we are beginning to see movement in the yoga community toward more robust standards of competence that are supported by both the received wisdom of tradition and emerging insights from multiple fields such as ayurveda (the science of life that is very much evolving), kinesiology, psychology, and neuroscience.

What does this mean for yoga teachers in the twenty-first century? As we started this story a few hundred pages back, there is no end to what we can learn. If, as a community of yoga teachers, we are committed to elevating the yoga teaching profession to a place of esteemed recognition and legitimacy, we must continue to raise our own standards. The two-hundred-hour minimum standard for yoga teacher training is likely to be increasingly seen as the bare minimum in preparing teachers to teach with the knowledge and skill required for basic competence, as are the ten hours of annual continuing education required of teachers under existing Yoga Alliance standards. We can, and I think should, do far more to train, guide, and give ongoing support to new teachers. We should also ask even the most experienced teachers to continue learning, to continue developing their skills and knowledge as the world of yoga continues to evolve and to be informed by advances across the arts and sciences of human development. Ensuring that students have teachers with comprehensive competence seems not like a lofty goal but rather the least we should promise.[7]

Now here you are. In every breath, you have the opportunity to consciously evolve as a teacher, a student, and a human. Breathe deeply to keep opening yourself to all the possibilities for how you can keep becoming the very best teacher you can be, one who recognizes and supports each and every student in discovering the best teacher they will ever have—the one dancing in their own heart.

Appendix B

Glossary

a: "Non-," as in *ahimsa*, "nonviolence."

abductor: Muscle that draws a bone away from the midline of the body.

adductor: Muscle that draws a bone toward the midline of the body.

adho: Downward.

adho mukha: Downward-facing.

afflictions: The five forms of suffering *(kleshas)*.

agni: Fire.

ahimsa: Nonviolence; not hurting.

ajna chakra: Third-eye chakra.

akarna: To the ear.

anahata chakra: Heart chakra.

ananda: Ecstasy; bliss; love.

anjali mudra: The gesture of *anjali*, palms together at the heart.

Anjaneya: The monkey god.

antara: Internal.

antara kumbhaka: Holding the breath after inhalation.

anterior: Forward; in front.

anuloma: With the grain. Refers to movement or breathing.

apana: Pelvis or lower abdomen.

Apanasana: Pelvic-floor poses; wind-relieving pose.

apana-vayu: Downward-moving *prana*.

aparigraha: Noncovoutness, one of the *yamas*.

ardha: Half.

asana: To take one's seat; a yoga pose; the third limb of ashtanga.

Astavakra: An Indian sage and Sanskrit scholar; the asana Astavakrasana, named for him.

asteya: Not stealing, one of the five *yamas*.

atman: The true self; consciousness.

aum: First described in the Upanishads as the originating and all-encompassing sound of the universe. Alternately spelled *om*.

avidya: Ignorance.

ayurveda: Ancient Indian "science of life"; traditional form of Indian medicine.

baddha: Bound.

bahya: External.

bahya kumbhaka: Suspension of the breath after complete exhalation.

baka: Crane.

bandha: To bind; energetic engagement.

bhadra: Peaceful or auspicious.

Bhagavad Gita: "Song of the Lord," a chapter in the epic Mahabharata and the most influential of all writings on yoga and spiritual philosophy.

bhakti: The practice of devotion.

Bharadvaj: An Indian sage.

Bharirava: An aspect of Shiva.

bhastrika: Bellows used in a furnace; type of *pranayama* where air is forcibly drawn in and out through the nostrils.

bhaya: Fear.

bheka: Frog.

bhuja: Arm or shoulder.

bhujanga: Cobra.

bhujapida: Pressure on the arm or shoulder.

Brahma: God; the supreme being; the creator; the first deity of the Hindu trinity.

brahmacharya: Celibacy; right use of sexual energy; one of the *yamas*.

brahman: Infinite consciousness.

buddhi: Intellect; seat of intelligence.

cervical spine: The vertebrae of the neck.

chakra: Subtle energy center.

chandra: Moon.

danda: Staff or stick.

dhanu: Bow.

dharana: Mental concentration; the sixth limb of Patanjali's ashtanga yoga.

dharma: Virtuous duty.

dhyana: Meditation.

dristi: Gazing point.

dukha: Pain; sorrow; grief.

dwi: Two.

eka: One.

ekagrata: One-pointed mental focus.

eka pada: One-legged or one-footed.

embody: Be an expression of or give a tangible or visible form to (an idea, quality, or feeling).

extension: Movement of a joint whereby one part of the body is moved away from another.

flexion: Bending movement that decreases the angle between two points.

Galava: An Indian sage.

garuda: Eagle; name of the king of birds. Garuda is represented as a vehicle of Vishnu and as having a white face, an aquiline beak, red wings, and a golden body.

Gheranda: A sage, the author of the Gheranda Samhita, a classical work on Hatha yoga.

gomukha: Cow head.

guna: Literally "rope," it refers to something that binds; in reference to yoga, it refers to the three intertwined fundamental properties inherent in all phenomena: *sattva, rajas,* and *tamas.*

guru: A spiritual preceptor, one who illuminates the spiritual path; alternately, you are you.

hala: Plough.

Hanuman: A monkey god, son of Anjaneya and Vayu.

hasta: Hand or arm.

Hatha yoga: Literally "forceful"; physical purification practices first described in written form in the fourteenth century CE in the Hatha Yoga Pradipika.

humerus: Upper arm bone.

hyperextension: Extension of a joint beyond 180 degrees.

ida: A *nadi* or channel of energy starting from the left nostril, moving to the crown of the head, and descending to the base of the spine.

insertion of muscles: End of the muscles that is distant from the center of the body.

Ishvara: The supreme being; Brahma with form.

isometric exercise: Exercise in which the muscles do not get shortened.

isotonic exercise: Exercise that involves shortening of a muscle.

jalandhara bandha: The chin lock where the chin is drawn toward the collarbones.

janu: Knee.

jathara: Belly.

jnana: Sacred knowledge derived from meditation on higher truths of religion and philosophy, which teaches people how to understand their own nature.

kapala: Skull.

kapalabhati: Skull cleansing, a *pranayama* technique.

kapha: One of the three ayurvedic humors.

kapota: Pigeon; dove.

karma: Action.

karma yoga: The yoga of action.

karna: Ear.

karnapida: Ears squeezed.

klesha: Suffering due to ignorance, egoism, desire, hatred, or fear.

kona: Angle.

Koundinya: A sage.

krama: Sequence of moments; succession of moments; stage.

Krishna: An incarnation of Vishnu; a form of God.

kriya: Action; also various purification practices.

krouncha: Heron.

kukkuta: Rooster.

kumbhaka: Breath retention after a complete inhalation or exhalation.

kundalini: Pranic energy, symbolized as a coiled and sleeping serpent lying dormant in the lowest nerve center at the base of the spinal column; a form of Hatha yoga practice.

kurma: Turtle.

kyphosis: Forward curvature of the spine.

laghu: Simple; little; small; handsome.

lateral: Sideways; away from the midline of the body.

lateral rotation: See *external rotation*.

laya: To merge.

lola: To swing or dangle.

lordosis: Backward curvature of the spine.

lumbar spine: The vertebrae of the lower back.

mahabandha: The great lock.

Mahabharata: A major Sanskrit epic of ancient India; contains the Bhagavad Gita and major elements of Hindu mythology.

maha mudra: The great seal.

mala: Garland, wreath.

mandala: Spiritually significant concentric form used for meditation and rituals.

manduka: Frog.

manipura chakra: Navel chakra.

manos: The individual mind.

mantra: Sacred sound, thought, or prayer.

Marichi: Name of a sage who is one of the sons of Brahma.

Matsyendra: Lord of the fishes; a tantric adept.

mayura: Peacock.

medial: Toward the midline of the body.

medial rotation: See *internal rotation*.

moksha: Liberation.

mudra: Seal; hand and finger positions or a specific combination of *asana, pranayama*, and *bandha*.

mukha: Face.

mula: Root, base.

mula bandha: Root lock; energetic engagement; sustained lifting of the perineum and levator ani.

muladhara chakra: Root chakra.

nadi: Literally "river"; energy channel.

nadi shodhana: Purification or cleansing of the *nadis; pranayama* technique for this purpose.

nakra: Crocodile.

namaskara: Salutation; greeting.

nara: Man.

naravirala: Sphinx.

Nataraja: Dancing Shiva.

nauli: Physical purification technique involving churning the belly.

nava: Boat.

nidra: Sleep.

niyama: Second limb of Patanjali's eight-limbed path; consists of *saucha, santosa, tapas, svadhyaya,* and *ishvarapranidhana.*

origin of a muscle: End of a muscle that is closer to the body center.

pada: Foot or leg.

pada hasta: Hands to feet.

padangustha: Big toe.

padma: Lotus.

parigha: Gate.

parigraha: Hoarding.

parinamavada: The constancy of change.

paripurna: Full.

parivrtta: Crossed; with a twist.

parsva: Side; flank; lateral.

paschimo: West; the back side of the body.

phalaka: Plank.

pincha: Chin; feather.

pinda: Fetus or embryo; body.

pingala: A *nadi* or channel or energy starting from the right nostril, moving to the crown of the head and downward to the base of the spine.

pitta: One of the three ayurvedic humors, sometimes translated as "bile."

posterior: Backward; opposite of *anterior.*

prakriti: Nature; the original source of the material world, consisting of *sattva, rajas,* and *tamas.*

prana: Life force; sometimes refers to the breath.

pranayama: Breath control; breath expansion; the fourth limb of ashtanga.

prasarana: Sweeping movement of the arms.

prasarita: Spread out; stretched out.

prasvasa: Expiration.

pratikriyasana: Counterpose.

pratiloma: Against the hair; against the grain.

pratyahara: Independence of the mind from sensory stimulation; the fifth stage of ashtanga.

prishta: Back.

puraka: Inhalation.

purna: Complete.

pursvo: East; the front of the body.

pursvottana: The intense stretch of the front side of the body.

raga: Love; passion; anger.

raja: King; ruler.

raja kapota: King pigeon.

rajas: Impulsive or chaotic thought; the aspect of movement in nature; one of the three *gunas.*

rechaka: Exhalation; emptying of the lungs.

sadhana: Practice for achievement.

sahasrara chakra: Thousand-petaled lotus, located in the cerebral cavity.

sahita: Aided.

sahita kumbhaka: Intentional suspension of breath.

salabha: Locust.

salamba: With support.

sama: Equal; same.

samadhana: Mental peace.

samadhi: Bliss; meditative absorption.

samasthihi: A state of balance.

samskara: Subconscious imprint.

samyama: Combined application of *dharana, dhyana,* and *samadhi.*

santosa: Contentment.

sarvanga: The whole body.

sattva: Light/order; one of the three elements of *prakriti.*

sattya: Truth; one of the five *yamas.*

saucha: Purity; cleanliness.

sava: Corpse.

setu bandha: Bridge.

Shakti: Life force, *prana;* consort of Shiva.

shishula: Dolphin.

Shiva: A form of God in Hinduism; the destroyer of illusion.

simha: Lion.

sirsa: Head.

sitali: A cooling form of *pranayama.*

slumpasana: Habitual collapse of the heart center associated with lackadaisical slumping of the spine and torso.

sukham: Comfort; ease; pleasure.

supta: Supine; sleeping.

surya: The sun.

sushumna: Central energy channel, located in the spinal column.

svadhisthana chakra: Seat of vital force, situated above the organs of generation.

svana: Dog.

svasa: Inspiration.

Swatmarama: Author of the Hatha Yoga Pradipika, the original book on Hatha yoga.

tada: Mountain.

tamas: Dullness; inertia; ignorance; one of the three *gunas.*

tantra: The practice of using all energies, including the mundane, for spiritual awakening.

tapa: Austerity.

tapas: heat; burning effort that involves purification, self-discipline, and austerity.

thoracic spine: The vertebrae of the rib cage.

tibia: Shinbone.

tiriang mukha: Backward-facing.

tittibha: Firefly.

tola: Balance; scales.

tri: Three.

trikona: Triangle.

ubhaya: Both.

udana: A *prana vayu.*

uddiyana: Upward flying; a *bandha.*

uddiyana bandha: Drawing the lower abdominal core in and up.

ujjayi: Victorious.

ujjayi pranayama: Basic yogic breathing.

Upanishad: To sit down near; ancient philosophical texts considered an early source of Hinduism.

upavista: Seated with legs spread.

urdhva: Upward.

ustra: Camel.

utkata: Awkward; powerful; fierce.

utpluti: Lifting or pumping up.

uttana: Upright intense stretch.

Uttanasana: Forward bend.

utthita: Extended.

vajra: Thunderbolt.

vakra: Crooked.

Vasistha: A Vedic sage.

vata: One of the three ayurvedic humors, sometimes translated as "wind."

vayu: Wind; vital air current.

Vedanta: Literally "end of the Vedas"; the dominant Hindu philosophical tradition.

Vedas: Oldest sacred texts of humankind.

vidya: Knowledge; learning; lore; science.

viloma: Against the hair; against the order of things.

vinyasa: To place in a special way; the conscious connection of breath and movement.

viparita: Inverted; upside-down.

vira: Hero; brave.

Virabhadra: A warrior.

Vishnu: A primary form of God in Hinduism; governs preservation, balance, sustainability.

vishuddha chakra: Pure; situated in the pharyngeal region.

vrksa: Tree.

vrschika: Scorpion.

vyana: A *prana vayu*.

yama: Restraint; contain; the first of the eight limbs of ashtanga yoga.

yama: To contain; the first limb of ashtanga, consisting of *ahimsa, sattya, brahmacharya, aparigraha,* and *asteya.*

yoga: From the root *yuj,* meaning "to join," "to yoke," "to make whole."

yoga-robics: Physical routines utilizing yoga asanas for purely physical exercise.

Appendix C

Additional Resources

The Teaching Yoga Resource Center (http://markstephensyoga.com/resources /overview) provides a variety of resources for yoga teachers and teacher trainers: teacher-training curriculum guides, instructional videos, audio recordings, articles, inspirational poetry, teacher-training program listings, and links to other resources.

Teaching Yoga: Essential Foundations and Techniques

Teaching Yoga is an essential resource for all yoga teachers and students interested in refining their skills and expanding their knowledge of yoga. Enhanced with over two hundred instructional photos and illustrations, this comprehensive book is ideal for use as a core textbook in teacher-training programs or for anyone interested in refining their understanding of the art and science of teaching yoga. Readers will find practical and detailed information on teaching methods, sequencing principles, the fundamentals of 108 asanas, and techniques for teaching pranayama and meditation. Yoga history and philosophy as well as traditional and modern aspects of anatomy are introduced, plus readers will find guidance on sustaining themselves as professional yoga teachers.

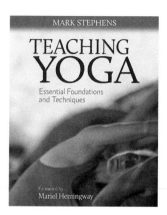

Yoga Sequencing: Designing Transformative Yoga Classes

The definitive resource for planning and sequencing safe, accessible, and sustainable yoga classes, *Yoga Sequencing* first presents a framework for thinking about sequencing through consideration of the philosophy, history, principles, and methods for approaching yoga. Yoga sequencing presents sixty-seven model sequences of yoga asanas that cover the broad range of yoga student experience, including multiple sequences for beginning, intermediate, and advanced students; yoga for kids, teens, women across the life cycle, and seniors; classes to relieve anxiety and depression; and sequences for each of the major chakras and ayurvedic constitutions. With over two thousand photos, this essential reference also explores the nuanced interrelationships among asanas within and among the seven asana families as well as how to sequence one's instructional cues, and it includes a useful appendix with valuable tools for planning one's own yoga practice or classes.

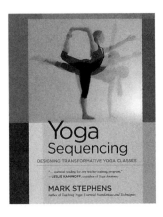

NOTES

Preface

1. See www.cpsc.gov/Research—Statistics/NEISS-Injury-Data.

2. See "In Over Their Heads," *Los Angeles Times,* August 13, 2001; Paul, "When Yoga Hurts," *Time,* October 4, 2007; Y. J. Krucoff (2003); Fishman and Saltonstall (2008); and Bertschinger et al. (2007). In my written reply to Broad, I emphasized that yoga is not a thing that can do something to you (a formulation that reifies yoga); rather, it is a practice the effects of which depend on one's condition, what one is doing, and how one is doing it. See Stephens (2012a).

Chapter 1: Philosophy and Sensibility in Giving Yoga Adjustments

1. Throughout this book we use the neologism *bodymind* in keeping with the view that the body and mind are not separate but rather a whole—and that sensing this whole is at the heart of yoga practice. This view stands in contrast to the dominant dualist views found in both Eastern and Western philosophy and forms a central theme of this book, which is primarily concerned with offering guidance to students that might help them more easily cultivate clear awareness of the wholeness of their being while in keeping with whatever intention motivates their yoga practice. This point is further explored later in this chapter.

2. Yoga originated in a culture rich in diverse spiritual and cultural practices and most significantly in Hindu-related belief, including Samkhya philosophy, but is neither reducible to nor necessarily bound to any particular belief system or religion. Such ties are a matter of choice. To explore further, see Devi (1960), Eliade (1969), Feuerstein (2001), Freeman (2012), Gates (2006), B. K. S. Iyengar (1966), Kempton (2013), Kramer and Alstad (1993), Rea (2013), Rosen (2012), Scaravelli (1991), Stephens (2010), Stryker (2011), David Gordon White (2011), and Ganga White (2007).

3. Some might object to applying the ideas of Western philosophical traditions to practices arising largely from Eastern philosophy and metaphysics. Here we take the view that any and all sources of insight should be considered, even if

we might disagree with certain concepts, propositions, or perspectives. Diverse sources of insight are thus incorporated throughout this book, even if from outside the normative or traditional purview of yoga.

4. For more on the fundamentals of sharing yoga, see Cope (2006), Farhi (2006), B. K. S. Iyengar (2009), Lasater (2009), Stephens (2010 and 2012a), Ganga White (2007), and Yogananda (1946).

5. Bikram Choudhury leads the way with competitive yoga, including current efforts to establish yoga as an Olympic sport. This is a curious phenomenon only if one ignores the origin of his yoga style in India's competitive body-building culture rather than believing his assertion that his style—and only his style—is the true expression of Patanjali's synthesis of yoga philosophy and method, which he either fails to understand or willfully distorts. See Choudhury (2000). On oxymoronic competitive yoga, see Lorr (2012) and the International Yoga Sports Federation (http://yogasportsfederation.org). On the proliferation of injuries when approaching yoga competitively, see Broad (2013).

6. Hatha yoga is the umbrella over all so-called "styles," "lineages," and brands of yoga in which postural practices are an integral element, from Ashtanga Vinyasa and Bikram to Iyengar and Power and hundreds of others. Note that the term *hatha* means "forceful," referring to the deliberate exertion one makes "in the service of transformation" (Rosen 2012, 7–8). For more on the origins and historical development of modern postural practices, see Rosen (2012), Singleton (2010), and David Gordon White (1996, 2003, and 2011). There is a reactive movement against this scholarship that is characterized by loose standards of veracity and unsubstantiated assertion in which even the slight suggestive piece of ancient iconography is claimed to confirm continuity of practice since the origins of yoga three thousand or more years ago. Such arguments are usually made in support of some notion of orthopraxy or yoga theology that bolsters the claim of a brand, lineage, or style of practice as being superior to or more legitimate than others.

7. Certainly, asana practice creates portals of insight into the truth of one's being, and as such is a potential meditation practice in itself and definitely a source of stability and ease in sitting meditation.

8. This approach is given further and refined explication by Ganga White (2007) as "surfing the edge" and Schiffmann (1996). See Stephens (2010) on applying this technique in teaching yoga.

9. For an insightful discussion of this deficit in today's classes, see Rosen (2012). Note that the Hatha Yoga Pradipika mostly addresses pranayama, not asana, which is only about ten percent of the book.

10. On sequentially introducing and teaching pranayamas, see Holleman and Sen-Gupta (1999, 267–92), B. K. S. Iyengar (1985), Rosen (2002 and 2006), and Stephens (2010, 237–62).

11. To learn more, see Stephens (2012b) on the philosophy, principles, and techniques of sequencing.

12. There is extensive research on the relationship among touch, awareness, meaning, emotional development, cognitive development, and consciousness. A good starting place for exploring is the work in Matthew Hertenstein's Touch and Emotion Lab at DePauw University. See Hertenstein (2011) on the communicative functions of touch in adulthood. See Field et al. (1997, 65–69), Field (2003), and Levine (2010) regarding touch with children and those with emotional trauma.

13. The role of the teacher is seen in vastly different ways depending on one's more general perspective on yoga, teaching, learning, pedagogy, and gurus. On teaching yoga, see Lasater (2000), Farhi (2006), and Stephens (2010). On pedagogy, see Bruner (1960) and Freire (1970). On gurus, see Cope (1999), Kramer and Alstad (1993), and Yogananda (1946).

14. This plays on a point made by Judith Lasater (2000) that among "the most important imperatives" for yoga teachers is that we are teaching people, not asanas, and that "each person is an individual to be taught, not a 'posture' to be fixed."

15. Levine (2010), Emerson and Hopper (2011).

16. There are many wonderful translations and interpretations of the Bhagavad Gita. My favorite basic translation is Prabhavananda and Isherwood (1944). For a work that brilliantly brings the messages of the Gita to practical life in contemporary experience, see Cope (2012).

17. See Diogenes (2000, 91, 95).

18. Certainly in Cartesian, Kantian, and Hegelian forms of philosophical dualism that guarantee conceptual space for the authority of religious doctrine and social forces that typically denigrate the body, much as in renunciate forms of fundamentalist yoga.

19. See Shusterman (2008) for an insightful discussion of how Dewey's work rescues analytical philosophy and phenomenology from dualism through the principles of mindfulness and somaesthetics. For a brilliant discussion of embodied habit and its effects on and expression in posture, emotion, and thought, see the pioneering work of Todd (1937).

20. Mihaly Csikszentmihalki (1990 and 1997) offers insights into how these qualities of being in everyday engagement in the flow of life generate deeper happiness through mindful challenge.

21. For a general introduction to somatics, see Hanna (2004). For practices of embodiment, see Don Hanlon Johnson (1995). For an anthology on body, breath, and consciousness, see Macnaughton (2004); also see Lakoff and Johnson (1999).

22. The Yoga Sutras of Patanjali are from around 200 CE. There are numerous and often contradictory translations and transliterations. The earliest writings on Hatha yoga date to a little over a thousand years later. See Bouanchaud (1999), B. K. S. Iyengar (2001), Kissiah (2011), Remski (2012), and Satchidananda (1978) for contrasting interpretations.

23. On sociocultural conditioning, see Durkheim (1912), Geertz (1973), and George Herbert Mead (1934).

24. Proprioceptive and kinesthetic awareness are at the heart of asana practice. Our proprioceptive awareness arises through dialogue between sensory neurons in muscle fiber (muscle spindle nerves) and the inner ear, creating a cognitive experience of balance and where one is in space. Our kinesthetic awareness arises from our proprioceptive awareness and manifests as we create movement in space with intentional behavior. Much of the refinement we cultivate in asana practice develops and refines these qualities of embodiment.

25. As Hertenstein (2011) discusses, touch is taboo in much of contemporary society, with detrimental effects on our lives.

26. On trauma, touch, and healing in yoga, see Emerson and Hopper (2011). Also see Cope (2006). On yoga therapy and more generally on healing, see Kraftsow (1995), Lasater (1995), McCall (2007), and Mohan and Mohan (2004). On the ethics of touch more generally, see Benjamin and Sohnen-Moe (2003).

Chapter 2: The Seven Principles of Hands-On Teaching

1. To learn functional anatomy, start by completing Kapit and Elson (2001). Learn more with Aldous (2004), Calais-Germain (1991), Kaminoff and Matthews (2011), Lasater (2009), Long (2009 and 2010), Moore and Dalley (1999), and Netter (1997).

2. See Diversity Council (2008) for a useful general guide to the areas of sensitivity one should respect in cross-cultural interaction. On gender and status patterns, see Major et al. (1990, 634–43) and Margaret Mead (1935). On the genetic effects of touch, see Schanberg (1995, 211–29). On touch in general, see Ackerman (1990), Field (2001), and Montagu (1986). On cross-species touch that is no less insightful in human interaction, see Haraway (2008).

3. See Lasater (2009) for a general discussion of active versus passive joint movement in the context of doing yoga asana. Lasater generally discourages passive joint movement.

4. On biomechanics and structural kinesiology, see Floyd (2006).

5. See Stephens (2010, 157–235) for basic alignment and energetic actions in each of 108 asanas.

Chapter 9: Seated and Supine Forward Bends and Hip Openers

1. All forward bends are hip openers, and many hip openers are forward bends. The classification of some asanas into one or the other asana family is thus somewhat arbitrary. For example, Upavista Konasana (Wide-Angle Forward Fold Pose) is clearly a hip-opening forward fold and a forward-folding hip opener. Here we treat them as being in one family.

Chapter 11: Guiding Yoga in the Twenty-First Century

1. To explore the scholarly literature on these questions, consider starting with Feuerstein (2001), Rosen (2012), Singleton (2010), Sjoman (1996), and David Gordon White (1996, 2000, 2003, 2011).

2. We find clear examples of yoga creation myths in the fantasy histories given by the gurus of Ashtanga Vinyasa (various stories, including direct transmission from the ninth-century sage Nathamuni to Tiramulai Krishnamacharya in the 1910s), Bikram (who says the asanas he teaches were "set down by Patanjali over four thousand years ago"), Tri-Yoga (founder Kali Ray's claim that she receives her teachings through direct transmission from ancient Kundalini *siddis*), Universal Free Style Yoga (Andrey Lappa's claim of direct transmission from the deity Shiva), and many others. See Desikachar (1995, 80–82), Choudhury (2000, xi), Ray (2013), and Lappa (2013).

3. Varene (1977, 226), Lowitz (2004, 85), Barnhart (1988, 447).

4. This and other testimonials from the disciples of various gurus are posted on www.writespirit.net/spirituality/gurus/benefits-guru.

5. To explore further, see Kramer and Alstad (1993), Preece (2010), and Krishnamurti (1987).

6. The evolutions we are presently witnessing in the yoga world relate to practically every aspect of human experience. For some of the more innovative and relevant examples, see Horton and Harvey (2012), and the various studies being conducted in conjunction with Stephen Cope's Institute for Extraordinary Living based at Kripalu Center for Yoga and Health (www.kripalu.org).

7. As this book goes to press, the author is working with eight others drawn from across North America on the Yoga Alliance Standards Working Group, with the task of making the standards clearer, stronger, and more accountable. To learn more about this work, visit www.yogaalliance.org.

REFERENCES

Ackerman, Diane. 1990. *A Natural History of the Senses.* New York: Random House.

Aldous, Susi Hately. 2004. *Anatomy and Asana: Preventing Yoga Injuries.* Calgary: Functional Synergy.

Alter, Michael J. 1996. *Science of Flexibility,* 2nd ed. Champaign, IL: Human Kinetics.

Avalon, Arthur. 1974. *The Serpent Power: Being the Sat-Cakra-Nirupana and Paduka-Pancaka.* New York: Dover.

Balaskas, Janet. 1994. Preparing for *Birth* with *Yoga.* Boston: Element.

Bandy, William D., and Jean M. Irion. 1994. "The Effect of Time on Static Stretch on the Flexibility of the Hamstring Muscles." *Physical Therapy* 74(9): 845–50.

Baptiste, Baron. 2003. *Journey into Power: How to Sculpt Your Ideal Body, Free Your True Self, and Transform Your Life with Yoga.* New York: Fireside.

Barnhart, Robert K. 1988. *The Barnhart Dictionary of Etymology.* New York: H. W. Wilson Co.

Benagh, Barbara. 2003. "Inversions and Menstruation." *Yoga Journal,* http://yogajournal.com/practice/546_1.cfm.

Benjamin, Ben E., and Cherie Sohnen-Moe. 2003. *The Ethics of Touch: The Hands-On Practitioner's Guide to Creating a Professional, Safe and Enduring Practice.* Tuscon: SMA Inc.

Bertschinger, Dimiter Robert, Efstratios Mendrinos, and André Dosso. 2007. "Yoga Can Be Dangerous–Glaucomatous Visual Field Defect Worsening Due to Postural Yoga." *British Journal of Ophthalmology* 91(1):1413–14, http://www.ncbi.nlm.nih.gov/pmc/articles/PMC2000997/.

Birch, Beryl Bender. 1995. *Power Yoga: The Total Strength and Flexibility Workout.* New York: Fireside.

———. 2000. *Beyond Power Yoga: 8 Levels of Practice for Body and Soul.* New York: Fireside.

Bouanchaud, Bernard. 1999. *The Essence of Yoga: Reflections on the Yoga Sutras of Patanjali.* New York: Sterling.

Briggs, Tony. 2001. "The Gift of Assisting." *Yoga Journal,* www.yogajournal.com/for_teachers/1024.

Broad, William J. 2013. *The Science of Yoga: The Risks and the Rewards*. New York: Simon and Schuster.

Bruner, Jerome. 1960. *The Process of Education*. Boston: Harvard University Press.

Calais-Germain, Blandine. 1991. *Anatomy of Movement*. Seattle: Eastland.

———. 2003. *The Female Pelvis: Anatomy and Exercises*. Seattle: Eastland.

———. 2005. *Anatomy of Breathing*. Seattle: Eastland.

Campbell, Joseph. 1949. *The Hero with a Thousand Faces*. New York: Pantheon.

Chinmayananda, Swami. 1987. *Glory of Ganesha*. Bombay: Central Chinmaya Mission Trust.

Choudhury, Bikram. 2000. *Bikram's Beginning Yoga Class*. New York: Penguin Putnam.

Clennell, Bobby. 2007. *The Woman's Yoga Book: Asana and Pranayama for All Phases of the Menstrual Cycle*. Berkeley, CA: Rodmell.

Cole, Roger. 2005. "With a Twist." *Yoga Journal* (November 2005).

———. 2006. "Protect the Knees in Lotus and Related Postures." *Yoga Journal*, www.yogajournal.com/for_teachers/978.

Cope, Stephen. 1999. *Yoga and the Quest for the True Self*. New York: Bantam.

———. 2006. *The Wisdom of Yoga: A Seeker's Guide to Extraordinary Living*. New York: Bantam-Bell.

———. 2012. *The Great Work of Your Life: A Guide for the Journey to Your True Calling*. New York: Bantam.

Csikszentmihalki, Mihaly. 1990. *Flow: The Psychology of Optimal Experience*. New York: Harper and Row.

———. 1997. *Creativity: Flow and the Psychology of Discovery and Invention*. New York: Harper Collins.

Desikachar, T. K. V. 1995. *The Heart of Yoga: Developing a Personal Practice*. Rochester, VT: Inner Traditions.

———. 1998. *Health, Healing, and Beyond: Yoga and the Living Tradition of Krishnamacharya*. New York: Aperture.

Devereux, Godfrey. 1998. *Dynamic Yoga: The Ultimate Workout That Chills Your Mind as It Charges Your Body*. New York: Thorsons.

Devi, Indra. 1960. *Yoga and You: A Complete 6 Weeks' Course for Home Practice*. Preston, UK: A. Thomas & Co.

Dewey, John, and Jo Ann Boydston. 2008a. *The Later Works, 1925–1953*. Carbondale, IL: Southern Illinois University Press.

———. 2008b. *The Middle Works, 1899–1924*. Carbondale, IL: Southern Illinois University Press.

Diogenes Laertius. 2000. *Lives of Eminent Philosophers*, Vol. 1. Boston: Loeb Classical Library.

Diversity Council. 2008. *Cross-Cultural Communication:*
Translating Nonverbal Cues, www.diversitycouncil.org/toolkit/Resources
_TipSheet_NonverbalCrossCulturalCOmmunication.pdf.

Durkheim, Émile. 1912. *The Elementary Forms of the Religious Life.* London: G. Allen
and Unwin.

Eliade, Mircea. 1969. *Yoga: Immortality and Freedom.* New York: Pantheon.

Emerson, David, and Elizabeth Hopper. 2011. *Overcoming Trauma through Yoga.*
Berkeley, CA: North Atlantic Books.

Espinoza, Fernando. 2005. "An Analysis of the Historical Development of Ideas about
Motion and Its Implications for Teaching." *Physical Education* 40(2).

Farhi, Donna. 1996. *The Breathing Book: Good Health and Vitality through Essential
Breath Work.* New York: Henry Holt.

———. 2006. *Teaching yoga: Exploring the Teacher-Student Relationship.* Berkeley,
CA: Rodmell Press.

Feuerstein, Georg. 2001. *The Yoga Tradition: Its History, Literature, Philosophy and
Practice.* Prescott, AZ: Hohm Press.

Field, Tiffany. 2001. *Touch.* Cambridge, MA: MIT Press.

———. 2003. *Touch Therapy.* Philadelphia: Churchill Livingstone.

Field, Tiffany, Maria Hernandez-Reif, Sybil Hart, Olga Quintino, Levelle A. Drose,
and Tory Field. 1997. "Effects of Sexual Abuse Are Lessened by Massage Therapy."
Journal of Bodywork and Movement Therapies 1:2, 65–69.

Finger, Alan. 2005. *Chakra Yoga: Balancing Energy for Physical, Spiritual, and Mental
Well-Being.* Boston: Shambhala.

Fishman, Loren, and Ellen Saltonstall. 2008. *Yoga for Arthritis.* New York: W. W.
Norton.

———. 2010. *Yoga for Osteoporosis.* New York: W. W. Norton.

Floyd, R. T. 2006. *Manual of Structural Kinesiology,* 17th ed. New York: McGraw-Hill.

Frawley, David. 1999. *Yoga and Ayurveda: Self-Healing and Self-Realization.* Twin
Lakes, WI: Lotus.

Freedman, Françoise Barbira. 2004. *Yoga for Pregnancy, Birth and Beyond.* New York:
Dorling Kindersley.

Freeman, Richard. 2012. *The Mirror of Yoga: Awakening the Intelligence of Body and
Mind.* Boston: Shambhala.

Freire, Paulo. 1970. *Pedagogy of the Oppressed.* New York: Herder and Herder.

French, Roger Kenneth. 2003. *Medicine before Science: The Rational and Learned
Doctor from the Middle Ages to the Enlightenment.* Cambridge, UK: Cambridge
University Press.

Friend, John. 2006. *Anusara Yoga Teacher Training Manual,* 9th ed. Woodlands, TX:
Anusara.

Gambhirananda, Swami. 1989. *Taittiriya Upanishad*. Calcutta: Advaita Ashram.

Gannon, Sharon, and David Life. 2013. *Yoga Assisting: A Complete Visual and Inspirational Guide to Yoga Asana Assists*. Self-published: Premier Digital Publishing.

Gardner, Howard. 1993. *Frames of Mind: The Theory of Multiple Intelligences*. New York: Basic.

Gaskin, Ina May. 2003. *Ina May's Guide to Childbirth*. New York: Bantam.

Gates, Janice. 2006. *Yogini: The Power of Women in Yoga*. San Rafael, CA: Mandala.

Geertz, Clifford. 1973. *The Interpretation of Cultures*. New York: Basic.

Grimes, John. 1996. *A Concise Dictionary of Indian Philosophy: Sanskrit Terms Defined in English*. New York: SUNY Press.

Gudmestad, Julie. 2003. "Let's Twist Again." *Yoga Journal* (January-February 2003).

Hanna, Thomas. 2004. *Somatics: Reawakening the Mind's Control of Movement, Flexibility, and Health*. Cambridge, MA: Da Capo Press.

Haraway, Donna. 2008. *When Species Meet*. Minneapolis: University of Minneapolis Press.

Hardy, L., R. Lye, and A. Heathcote. 1983. "Active Versus Passive Warm-Up Regimes and Flexibility." *Research Papers in Physical Education* 1:5, 23–30.

Hertenstein, Matthew, ed. 2011. *The Handbook of Touch: Neuroscience, Behavioral, and Health Perspectives*. New York: Springer.

Hirschi, Gertrud. 2000. *Mudras: Yoga in Your Hands*. Boston: Weiser.

Hittleman, Richard. 1982. *Richard Hittleman's Yoga: 28-Day Exercise Plan*. New York: Bantam.

Holleman, Dona, and Orit Sen-Gupta. 1999. *Dancing the Body Light: The Future of Yoga*. Amsterdam: Pandion.

Horton, Carol, and Roseanne Harvey, eds. 2012. *21st-Century Yoga: Culture, Politics, and Practice*. Chicago: Kleio.

Iyengar, B. K. S. 1966. *Light on Yoga*. New York: Schockten.

———. 1985. *Light on Pranayama: The Yogic Art of Breathing*. New York: Crossroad.

———. 1988. *The Tree of Yoga*. Boston: Shambhala.

———. 2001. *Yoga: The Path to Holistic Health*. London: Dorling Kindersley.

———. 2009. *Yoga Wisdom and Practice*. London: Dorling Kindersley.

Iyengar, Geeta S. 1995. *Yoga: A Gem for Women*. Spokane: Timeless.

James, William. 1890. *The Principles of Psychology*. New York: H. Holt and Co.

———. 1976. *Essays in Radical Empiricism*. Cambridge, MA: Harvard University Press.

Johari, Harish. 1987. *Chakras: Energy Centers of Transformation*. Rochester, VT: Destiny.

Johnson, Don Hanlon, ed. 1995. *Bone, Breath, and Gesture: Practices of Embodiment.* Berkeley, CA: North Atlantic Books.

Johnson. Mark. 1989. *The Meaning of the Body: Aesthetics of Human Understanding.* Chicago: University of Chicago Press.

———. 1995. *The Body in the Mind: The Bodily Basis of Meaning, Imagination, and Reason.* Chicago: University of Chicago Press.

Jois, Sri K. Pattabhi. 2002. *Yoga Mala.* New York: North Point.

Jung, Carl. 1953. "Yoga and the West." *The Collected Works of Carl Jung,* Vol. 1., edited by Herbert Read, Michael Fordham, and Gerard Adler. New York: Bollingen.

Kaminoff, Leslie, and Amy Matthews. 2011. *Yoga Anatomy,* 2nd ed. Champaign, IL: Human Kinetics.

Kapit, Wynn, and Lawrence Elson. 2001. *The Anatomy Coloring Book.* San Francisco: Benjamin Cummings.

Kapur, Kamla K. 2007. *Ganesha Goes to Lunch: Classics from Mystic India.* San Rafael, CA: Mandala.

Keedwell, Paul. 2008. *How Sadness Survived: The Evolutionary Basis of Depression.* Oxford, UK: Radcliffe.

Kempton, Sally. 2013. *Awakening Shakti: The Transformative Power of the Goddess in Yoga.* Boulder, CO: Sounds True.

Kissiah, Gary. 2011. *The Yoga Sutras of Patanjali: Illuminations through Image, Commentary, and Design.* Los Gatos, CA: Lilalabs.

Kraftsow, Gary. 1999. *Yoga for Wellness: Healing with the Timeless Teachings of Viniyoga.* New York: Penguin.

Kramer, Joel. 1977. "A New Look at Yoga: Playing the Edge of Mind and Body." *Yoga Journal* (January 1977).

———. 1980. "Yoga as Self-Transformation." *Yoga Journal* (May-June 1980).

Kramer, Joel, and Diana Alstad. 1993. *The Guru Papers.* Berkeley, CA: North Atlantic Books.

———. 2009. *The Passionate Mind Revisited: Expanding Personal and Social Awareness.* Berkeley, CA: North Atlantic Books.

Krishnamurti, Jiddu. 1987. *The Awakening of Intelligence.* New York: HarperCollins.

Krucoff, Carol. 2003. "Insight from Injury." *Yoga Journal,* http://www.yogajournal.com/lifestyle/908.

Lad, Vasant. 1984. *Ayurveda: The Science of Self-Healing.* Twin Lakes, WI: Lotus.

Lakoff, George, and Mark Johnson. 1999. *Philosophy in the Flesh: The Embodied Mind and Its Challenge to Western Thought.* New York: Basic.

Lappa, Andrey. 2013. "Andrey Lappa Bio," www.universal-yoga.com/?id=14501.

Lasater, Judith. 1995. *Relax and Renew: Restful Yoga for Stressful Times.* Berkeley, CA: Rodmell.

———. 2000. *Living Your Yoga: Finding the Spiritual in Everyday Life.* Berkeley, CA: Rodmell.

———. 2009. *Yoga Body: Anatomy, Kinesiology, and Asana.* Berkeley, CA: Rodmell.

Levine, Peter. 2010. *In an Unspoken Voice: How the Body Releases Trauma and Restores Goodness.* Berkeley, CA: North Atlantic Books.

Long, Ray. 2009. *The Key Muscles of Yoga: Scientific Keys,* Vol. I. Plattsburgh, NY: Bandha Yoga.

———. 2010. *The Key Poses of Yoga: Scientific Keys,* Vol. II. Plattsburgh, NY: Bandha Yoga.

Lorr, Benjamin. 2012. *Hell-Bent: Obsession, pain, and the Search for Something Like Transcendence in Competitive Yoga.* New York: St. Martin's Press.

Lowitz, Leza A. 2004. *Sacred Sanskrit Words.* Berkeley, CA: Stone Bridge.

Macnaughton, Ian. 2004. *Body, Breath, and Consciousness: A Somatics Anthology.* Berkeley, CA: North Atlantic Books.

Maehle, Gregor. 2006. *Ashtanga Yoga: Practice and Philosophy.* Novato, CA: New World Library.

Major, Brenda, Anne Marie Schmidlin, and Lynne Williams. 1990. "Gender Patterns in Social Touch: The Impact of Setting and Age." *Journal of Personality and Social Psychology* 58:4, 634–43.

Mallinson, James, trans. 2004. *The Gheranda Samhita.* Woodstock, NY: YogaVidya.com.

Manchester, Frederick. 2002. *The Upanishads: Breath of the Eternal.* New York: Signet Classics.

McCall, Timothy, 2007. *Yoga as Medicine: The Yogic Prescription for Health and Healing.* New York: Bantam Dell.

Mead, George Herbert. 1934. *Mind, Self, and Society: From the Standpoint of a Social Behaviorist.* Chicago: University of Chicago Press.

Mead, Margaret. 1935. *Sex and Temperament in Three Primitive Societies.* New York: Harper.

Merleau-Ponty, Maurice. 1958. *Phenomenology of Perception.* London: Routledge.

Miller, Elise Browning. 2003. *Yoga for Scoliosis.* Menlo Park, CA: self-published.

Mittelmark, Raul Artal, Robert A. Wiswell, and Barbara L. Drinkwater, eds. 1991. *Exercise in Pregnancy,* 2nd ed. Baltimore: Williams & Wilkins.

Mohan, A. G. 1993. *Yoga for Body, Breath, and Mind: A Guide to Personal Reintegration.* Portland, OR: Rudra.

Mohan, A. G., and Indra Mohan. 2004. *Yoga Therapy: A Guide to the Therapeutic Use of Yoga and Ayurveda for Health and Fitness.* Boston: Shambhala.

Montagu, Ashley. 1986. *Touching: The Human Significance of Skin.* New York: William Morrow.

Moore, Keith L., and Arthur F. Dalley. 1999. *Clinically Oriented Anatomy,* 4th ed. Baltimore: Lippincott Williams & Wilkins.

Muktibodhananda Saraswati. 1985. *Hatha Yoga Pradipika: The Light on Hatha Yoga.* Munger, India: Bihar School of Yoga.

Myers, Esther. 2002. *Hands-On Assisting: A Guide for Yoga Teachers.* Toronto: Explorations in Yoga.

Netter, Frank H. 1997. *Atlas of Human Anatomy,* 2nd ed. East Hanover, NJ: Novartis.

Pappas, Stephanie. 2006. *Yoga Posture Adjustments and Assisting: An Insightful Guide for Yoga Teachers and Students.* Somerset, NJ: Trafford.

Prabhavananda, Swami, and Christopher Isherwood, trans. 1944. *Bhagavad Gita.* Los Angeles: The Vedanta Society.

Preece, Rob. 2010. *The Wisdom of Imperfection: The Challenge of Individuation in Buddhist Life.* Ithaca, NY: Snow Lion.

Ray, Kali. 2013. "Yogini Kaliji, Founder of TriYoga," www.triyoga.com/Kali_Ray/kali _ray_founder_of_triyoga.php.

Rea, Shiva. 1997. *Hatha Yoga as a Practice of Embodiment.* Master's thesis, University of California, Los Angeles, World Arts and Cultures (Dance) Department.

————. 2013. *Tending the Heart Fire: Living in the Flow with the Pulse of Life.* Boulder, CO: Sounds True.

Remski, Matthew. 2012. *Threads of Yoga: A Remix of Patanjali's Sutras with Commentary and Reverie.* Self-published.

Rosen, Richard. 2002. *The Yoga of Breath: A Step-by-Step Guide to Pranayama.* Boston: Shambhala.

————. 2006. *Pranayama Beyond the Fundamentals: An In-Depth Guide to Yogic Breathing.* Boston: Shambhala.

————. 2012. *Original Yoga: Rediscovering Original Practices of Hatha Yoga.* Boston: Shambhala.

Satchidananda, Swami. 1970. *Integral Hatha Yoga.* Austin: Holt, Rinehart and Winston.

————, trans. 1978. *The Yoga Sutras of Patanjali.* Buckingham, VA: Integral Yoga.

Scaravelli, Vanda. 1991. *Awakening the Spine: The Stress-Free New Yoga That Works with the Body to Restore Health, Vitality and Energy.* New York: HarperCollins.

Schanberg, Saul. 1995. "Genetic Basis for Touch Effects." In *Touch in Early Development,* T. Field, ed. Mahwah, NJ: Lawrence Erlbaum Associates, 211–29.

Schatz, Mary Pullig. 2002. "A Woman's Balance: Inversions and Menstruation," www .iyengar.ch/Deutsch/text_menstruation.htm.

Schiffmann, Erich. 1996. *Yoga: The Spirit and Practice of Moving into Stillness.* New York: Pocket.

Shrier, Ian, and Kav Gossal. 2000. "The Myths and Truths of Stretching: Individualized Recommendations for Healthy Muscles." *Physician and Sportsmedicine* 28:8.

Shusterman, Richard. 2008. *Body Consciousness: A Philosophy of Mindfulness and Somaesthetics.* New York: Cambridge University Press.

———. 2012. *Thinking Through the Body: Essays in Somaesthetics.* New York: Cambridge University Press.Singer, Charles A. 1957. *A Short History of Anatomy and Physiology from the Greeks to Harvey.* New York: Dover.

Singleton, Mark. 2010. *Yoga Body: The Origins of Modern Postural Practice.* New York: Oxford University Press.

Sjoman, N. E. 1996. *The Yoga Tradition of the Mysore Palace.* New Delhi: Abhinav.

Stenhouse, Janita. 2001. *Sun Yoga: The Book of Surya Namaskar.* St-Christophe, France: Innerspace.

Stephens, Mark. 2010. *Teaching Yoga: Essential Foundations and Techniques.* Berkeley, CA: North Atlantic Books.

———. 2011a. "Art of Asana: Effort and Ease in Handstand." *Yoga International* 113.

———. 2011b. "Art of Asana: Divine Expression—the Path to Natarajasana." *Yoga International* 114.

———. 2012a. "How Yoga Will Not Wreck Your Body." *Elephant Journal,* www.elephantjournal.com/2012/01 /how-yoga-will-not-wreck-your-body-mark-stephens/.

———. 2012b. *Yoga Sequencing: Designing Transformative Yoga Classes.* Berkeley, CA: North Atlantic Books.

Stryker, Rod. 2011. *The Four Desires: Creating a Life of Purpose, Happiness, Prosperity, and Freedom.* New York: Delacorte.

Swatmarama, Swami. 2004. *Hatha Yoga Pradipika.* Woodstock, NY: YogaVidya.com.

Swenson, David. 1999. *Ashtanga Yoga: The Practice Manual.* Austin: Ashtanga Yoga Productions.

Tirtha, Swami Sada Shiva. 2006. *The Ayurvedic Encyclopedia.* Coconut Creek, FL: Educa.

Todd, Mabel. 1937. *The Thinking Body: A Study of the Balancing Forces of Dynamic Man.* Gouldsboro, ME: Gestalt Journal Press.

Varene, Jean. 1977. *Yoga and the Hindu Tradition.* Chicago: University of Chicago Press.

Vasu, Rai B. Chandra, trans. 2004. *The Siva Samhita.* New Delhi: Munshiram Manoharial.

Vaughan, Kathleen. 1951. *Exercises before Childbirth.* London: Faber.

Weintraub, Amy. 2004. *Yoga for Depression: A Compassionate Guide to Relieve Suffering through Yoga.* New York: Broadway.

White, David Gordon. 1996. *The Alchemical Body: Siddha Traditions in Medieval India.* Chicago: University of Chicago Press.

———, ed. 2000. *Tantra in Practice.* Princeton, NJ: Princeton University Press.

———. 2003. *Kiss of the Yogini: "Tantric Sex" in Its South Asian Contexts.* Chicago: University of Chicago Press.

———. 2009. *Sinister Yogis.* Chicago: University of Chicago Press.

———, ed. 2011. *Yoga in Practice.* Princeton, NJ: Princeton University Press.

White, Ganga. 2007. *Yoga beyond Belief: Insights to Awaken and Deepen Your Practice.* Berkeley, CA: North Atlantic Books.

Woolery, Allison, H. Myers, B. Sternlieb, and L. Zelter. 2004. "A Yoga Intervention for Young Adults with Elevated Symptoms of Depression." *Alternative Therapies in Health and Medicine* 10:2, 60–63.

Yogananda, Paramhansa. 1946. *Autobiography of a Yogi.* Los Angeles: Self-Realization Fellowship.

INDEX

Eka Pada Raj Kapotasana I (One-Leg
   King Pigeon Pose I)
   adjustments for, 281
   description of, 280
   modification of, 281–82
   pronunciation of, 322
   resources for, 282
Eka Pada Raj Kapotasana II (One-Leg
   King Pigeon Pose II)
   adjustments for, 205–6
   description of, 205
   modification of, 207
   pronunciation of, 322
   resources for, 207
Eka Pada Sirsasana (One Leg behind
   Head Pose)
   adjustments for, 283
   description of, 282
   pronunciation of, 322
   resources for, 284
   variation of, 284
Embryo Pose. *See* Pindasana
Energetic actions, 39
Extended Hand to Big Toe Pose. *See*
   Utthita Hasta Padangusthasana
Extended Leg Pose. *See* Uttana Padasana
Extended Side Angle Pose. *See* Utthita
   Parsvakonasana
Extended Triangle Pose. *See* Utthita
   Trikonasana

F

Farhi, Donna, 23
Feathered Peacock Pose. *See* Pincha
   Mayurasana
Feet, activation of, 74
Final Relaxation Pose. *See* Savasana
Finger Draw, 67
Finger Flicks, 67
Finger Spread, 66
Firefly Pose. *See* Tittibhasana
Fire Log Pose. *See* Agnistambhasana

Fish Pose. *See* Matsyasana
Flying Crow Pose. *See* Galavasana
Flying Fish Pose. *See* Uttana Padasana
Flying Lizard Pose. *See* Uttana
   Prasithasana
Forearm Balance. *See* Pincha
   Mayurasana
Forrest, Ana, 137
Forward bends, 241–42. *See also indi-*
   vidual asanas
Four-Limbed Staff Pose. *See* Chaturanga
   Dandasana
Friend, John, 22
Frog Pose. *See* Bhekasana
Full Boat Pose. *See* Paripurna Navasana

G

Galavasana (Flying Crow Pose)
   adjustments for, 179–80
   description of, 178–79
   pronunciation of, 323
   resources for, 180
   transitioning from, 182
Gardner, Howard, 11
Garland Pose. *See* Malasana
Garudasana (Eagle Pose)
   adjustments for, 133
   description of, 133
   hip abductors and, 243
   modification of, 134
   pronunciation of, 323
   resources for, 134
Garudasana Prep (Eagle Prep Pose)
   adjustments for, 132
   description of, 131
   resources for, 132
Gomukhasana (Cow Face Pose)
   adjustments for, 274–75
   description of, 274
   external rotators and, 243
   hip abductors and, 243
   modification of, 275

ABOUT THE AUTHOR

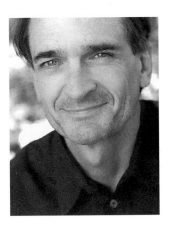

An esteemed yoga guide, author, and media producer who has trained over 1,200 yoga teachers, Mark Stephens conducts trainings, workshops, retreats, and classes worldwide. Practicing since 1991 and teaching since 1996, Stephens has explored diverse and complementary approaches along his path as student and teacher, including Ashtanga Vinyasa, Iyengar, Vinyasa Flow, yoga therapy, tantra, functional yoga anatomy and kinesiology, traditional yoga philosophies, and modern philosophies of being and consciousness. He lives and teaches in Santa Cruz, California, and directs the teacher-training program at Santa Cruz Yoga.

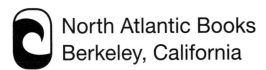

North Atlantic Books
Berkeley, California

Personal, spiritual, and planetary transformation

North Atlantic Books, a nonprofit publisher established in 1974, is dedicated to fostering community, education, and constructive dialogue. NABCommunities.com is a meeting place for an ever-growing membership of readers and authors to engage in the discussion of books and topics from North Atlantic's core publishing categories.

NAB Communities offer interactive social networks in these genres:

NOURISH: Raw Foods, Healthy Eating and Nutrition, All-Natural Recipes

WELLNESS: Holistic Health, Bodywork, Healing Therapies

WISDOM: New Consciousness, Spirituality, Self-Improvement

CULTURE: Literary Arts, Social Sciences, Lifestyle

BLUE SNAKE: Martial Arts History, Fighting Philosophy, Technique

Your free membership gives you access to:

Advance notice about new titles and exclusive giveaways

Podcasts, webinars, and events

Discussion forums

Polls, quizzes, and more!

Go to www.NABCommunities.com and join today.